How to Beat the Stress Epidemic

Mind/Body Strategies for Enhancing Well-Being

Éric Marlien DO, PT

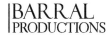

BARRAL
PRODUCTIONS

Palm Beach Gardens, FL

LCCN: 2017934436
ISBN-13: 978-0-9987479-0-3

Barral Productions
11211 Prosperity Farms Road, Suite D-325
Palm Beach Gardens, Florida 33410 USA
561.622.3761

Notice
Neither the Publisher nor the Authors assume any responsibility for any loss, injury and/or
damage to persons or property arising out of, or related to, any use of the material
contained in this book. It is the responsibility of the treating practitioner, relying on
independent expertise and knowledge of the patient, to determine the best treatment and
method of application for the patient.

The Publisher

Editors: Fred von Kamecke, Nathan Jacobs
Translator: Annabel Mackenzie RST, BI-D
Project Managers: Dawn Langnes Shear, Vicki McCabe
Artist: Jeri Monastero

**BARRAL
PRODUCTIONS**
Your source for quality educational materials.

www.Barralinstitute.com

Printed in the U.S.A.

CONTENTS

CONTENTS

Introduction

For whom is this book written?

For anyone who, in one way or another, feels their life is a succession of difficulties. These could be due to external stress linked to the ups and downs of daily life, which have intensified in modern times. Or they could be due to internal, psychological stress connected to their personal narratives, whose traces continue to torment in some way.

It is also written with therapists and health care professionals in mind. It focuses particularly on those seeking a reliable and comprehensive method of helping patients find lasting solutions to psychological and psychosomatic ills.

Stress has assumed "epidemic" proportions. Entering the word in a search engine turns up more than 42,500,000 responses in French alone, and over 581,000,000 worldwide.[1] With such numbers, it is difficult to predict whether an umpteenth book on the subject will find any readership, or simply pass unnoticed, like a strand of hair in a salon.

While there would appear to be no end of websites and books promoting an array of therapeutic or commercial solutions to "fighting stress," I am not discouraged for two reasons. The first is that I continue to meet patients in my clinical practice who not only suffer from stress, but are ill equipped to deal with it in a positive manner, avoid its psychosomatic consequences, or find a way to live in such a way that might limit it. All this despite an apparent deluge of information and solutions at their disposal.

[1] At the date of November 6, 2016.

The second is my intention to show that stress management, and, more broadly, the topic of emotional balance, cannot be understood from a single point of view. To this end, I have taken a multifaceted (scientific, psychological, and philosophical)—albeit simplified—approach, and proposed a series of practical solutions in line with these comprehensive considerations.

I will have achieved my goal if some people, as a result of this book, are able to find, or rediscover, some measure of control and serenity in their life. It is my wish that they become aware that reducing daily stress is an entirely personal process of shifting attitudes, and that it is up to us alone to exercise our freedom and creative power in every aspect of our existence.

The term "stress" is much overused nowadays and conceals more meaning than its banal usage implies. Reducing the word to a cliché leads to very inconsistent usage. Just saying the word stress can suggest we have some command over its causes and consequences, without taking the true measure of what it reveals about the human being who suffers. A person's history, family sociocultural conditioning, ontological, or neurophysiological functioning, not to mention the long-term implications for future health, are all involved.

Few solutions are offered to the stressed person. Doctors, friends, relatives, and therapists of all stripe, are often ineffectual, sometimes being themselves as stressed out as the patient. Either they do not know the appropriate solutions and steps to be implemented, or have not managed to put them into practice. In this, no one is to blame; as we shall see, real and effective solutions require a good deal more resolve than swallowing pills or going for an anti-stress massage. That may be pleasant enough, but of little preventive or curative value.

This book takes an interest in all these aspects, glancing over some and delving more deeply into others, in accordance with my knowledge and experience over the course of twenty years in professional practice. I will try to answer questions as clearly as possible, keeping in mind that no response can be definitive, and in the hope that the perspective presented gives rise to new discussion. This is how our collective understanding advances. The first part of the book is essentially theoretical. After a brief exploration of the stress phenomenon, the study of the autonomic nervous system features prominently. This division of the nervous system sits at the crossroads of the body and mind, regulating our stress response, as well as the ensuing disorders and illnesses that can result.

Cardiac coherence, a harmonious state where the heart and mind are united, is presented as a new approach to illness and health. It offers a practical synthesis of the theoretical knowledge provided in the preliminaries.

The second part of the book is devoted to practices that, far from being exhaustive or necessarily superior to other methods, have nevertheless, been found to be tried and true by countless people who use them every day. Exercises are organized around three axes: physiological, emotional, and mental. A balanced life requires that these functional components of the human personality be well-balanced, developed, and coordinated. Such harmony is the basis for optimal adaptability, and allows an individual to build a fuller and more creative existence.

This book presents to the reader reflections on our existence—organization, priorities, meaning, and all the elements that truly inform our way of dealing with or generating stress. The value that a human being gives to life and to himself, brings up questions that get to the heart of what is important in life. This seems to me, to be the key issue.

PART ONE

Theory

1 ⌒

What is stress?

On the mechanical level, stress denotes any pressure or tension from an external source. The agent of this pressure is the "stressor," and can be distinguished from the response to it, or what we call "stress."

Common usage confuses the terms stress and stressor. Stress is considered to be the interaction between the external cause and the resistance to it deployed by an organism in the form of external opposition or aggressive reaction.

When we bend a bow, for example, the action of one hand puts an external load on the string, while our other hand exerts a counter force on the bow itself. How a given bow responds to mechanical stress depends on its shape, size, pre-existing level of tension, as well as the material of which it is made. Whereas one bow might hardly bend, another could bend to the optimal level for launching an arrow, and yet a third would snap under the load.

Nature requires that human beings, indeed every living creature, be adaptable to all external force or stimulation received by the organism. Stimulation constitutes external force, in that it represents a degree of kinetic energy that affects living structures in such a way that they react by moving. This notion of movement can be expanded to include all manner of changes and variations.

Images that form instantaneously, even in our mind's eye, are the result of energy. Light is composed of photons that vary in wavelength, depending on the color of objects set before us. Light acts on specialized retinal cells that convert energy into force. These cells are the site of chemical and electrical activities that transmit to specialized visual centers in the cerebral cortex. Adaptation phenomena can be simple, involving only local reaction, or can be so complex as to mobilize the entire organism.

Upon entering a darkened room, for example, the dimness causes our pupils to widen in an effort to capture as much light as possible. Whereas they contract when we move from darkness to light. Imagine that you sense danger in a darkened place—the threat of a lion, for example—adaptations become immediately more complex. Glucose and adrenaline are discharged into the bloodstream, the heart rate accelerates, and blood is shunted away from the digestive organs to the muscles. A cascade of physiological events prepares you for fight or flight.

The human organism is perpetually subjected to stimulation of all sorts, the great majority of which rest below the threshold of conscious awareness. Our bodies continuously adapt to innumerable micro stresses by regulating variables, in order that internal conditions remain stable and relatively constant. This is called homeostasis.

Thought of in this way, stress is not in itself a pejorative, but rather an animating force between one system and another. Stress guarantees that nothing remains static in nature. By the same token stress is the source of all change, interrelationships, evolution, action, and eventual degradation.

Without "stress" placed on a bow, an arrow would never reach its target. This leads us to consider the classical division between pathological stress and normal stress, or what is termed "eustress."

Biological equilibrium and the rhythms of all living beings depend on a steady stream of influence that surrounds us from the first appearance of biological molecules at conception. The privation of these external influences—stressors that are also stimulants—invariably leads to the death of the organism. In other words, physiological stress is responsible for the maintenance of vital base tonus.

Whenever stress passes a certain arbitrary threshold, beyond which a given organism can effectively cope, stress assumes increasingly negative proportions, to the point of initiating an irreversible pathological condition, leading even to death. This is the last stage of adaptation, sometimes described as the final escape.

The endocrinologist Hans Selye defined stress as, "the non-specific response of the body to demands placed upon it."[1] The nature of the stress agent can be extraordinarily varied: physical, chemical, toxic, infectious, traumatic, as well as any event that cause an intense emotional reaction. It is impossible to be categorical when defining the elements of stress. In Selye's view, "stress factors are considered to be all things that provoke the response syndrome we call stress.[2]

Psycho-emotional stress is very often chronic in nature, rather than the result of a sudden intense or overwhelming event. A stable, outwardly peaceful situation may in fact be subjecting a person to ongoing strain, whose effect on internal equilibrium can be as fearsome as a violent shock. It is also evident that the effects of stress are much more harmful when the stress is perceived—in reality or just as a belief—as fatalistic and to be entirely beyond control.

We will see in this book that this personal aspect is the important variable. For it is here that rests the freedom and power of each individual. Our internal balance belongs to none other than ourselves. Our ability or inability to have some measure of control over events or our surroundings is often a belief deeply ingrained, rooted to our past conditioning.

For example, while it is entirely impossible for human beings to jump from a height of as much as fifty meters and survive, jumping just one meter might appear inordinately stressful to a person who believes that such an action might be dangerous. One individual might readily jump a meter, and another might feel coerced into the event and, not jumping of his own free

[1] Lôo, Pierre, Lôo Henri and Galinowski André, *Le stress permanent*, Masson, 1999, p.6.

[2] Millenson J. R., *Le corps et l'esprit*, DésIris, 1998, p.76.

will, be at greater risk of injury. The mechanical stress is the same in both cases, but the one who made his own choice amuses himself through the sheer pleasure of the jump.

2 ᴄᴄ

A Brief History
of Stress Research

A good deal of experimental research emerged in the twentieth century. Psychophysiological studies and theories followed an evolutionary perspective—the interpretation of how living creatures adapt to their environment.

Ivan Pavlov (1849-1936) is famous for his pioneering work on what he called the conditional reflex. According to Pavlov, "Man, like all animals, is continuously bombarded with information, in the form of excitation arising from both inside the body and the external world. The cortex analyzes the information and provides conditioned responses that allow the organism to adapt to his environment."[1] In the face of conflicting information, animals exhibit disturbed behavior, something Pavlov called "experimental neurosis." The Pavlovian school went on to show that biological phenomena can stem from emotional or mental states, including psychogenic disorders. Pavlov's work gave rise to modern behavioral therapy. It inspired ethology, the study of animal behavior, which is the foundation of cortico-visceral medicine, or the natural functional interaction between the cerebral cortex and the internal organs. The instigator was the physiologist Konstantin Bykov (1886-1959) who, with the help of his team, was able to prove that malignant tumors can develop in dogs submitted to long standing experimental neurosis.

---

[1] Kamieniecki, Hanna, *History of the Psychosomatic,* P.U.F., 1994, p.135.

Walter Cannon (1871-1945) wrote a classic treatise on homeostasis. He demonstrated the impact of emotions on hormone balance and other factors that regulate our internal environment. "For the first time, it was possible to experimentally reproduce visceral manifestation of emotion, and to understand how a mental state resounds within by the body."[2] Cannon was able to demonstrate that in an alarming or emotionally intense situation, the sympathetic nervous system initiates reaction in the body and the adrenal medulla releases a cascade of hormones

Hans Selye (1907-1982) was a pioneering endocrinologist who authored many research publications on the biological reaction of an organism to stressors. He named this response, the *general adaptation syndrome.*

Cannon and Selye's research shows linear causality:

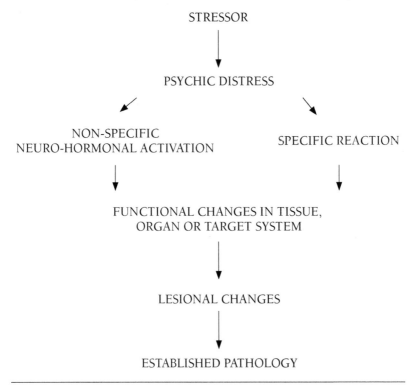

STRESSOR

PSYCHIC DISTRESS

NON-SPECIFIC
NEURO-HORMONAL ACTIVATION

SPECIFIC REACTION

FUNCTIONAL CHANGES IN TISSUE,
ORGAN OR TARGET SYSTEM

LESIONAL CHANGES

ESTABLISHED PATHOLOGY

---

[2] Dantzer, Robert, *The Psychosomatic Illusion,* Odile Jacob, 1989, p.22.

Physiologists consider a problem to be functional if the perceived threat is of low intensity and/or the distress that follows is of short duration. The problem can become a somatic dysfunction and organic pathology can manifest when the adaptive capacities are overwhelmed, as happens when the intensity of the stress agent and the stress responses becomes stronger or passes a certain threshold of duration.

Looking at the schematic above, one can see that our response options are essentially located at the level of "psychic distress." While it is possible to limit stress by living in a way that offers some protection, we are regularly buffeted by multiple and varied stressors.

How can we avoid succumbing to psychic distress, to transform our environment and our existence in such a way that habitual stressors are diminished and we can avoid subjecting our bodies to weakening imbalances? Such questions and solutions to them are explored in the pages to come.

Relative to the time and effort you have put in, do you feel that changes in the quality of your life, including the benefits to physiological, emotional, and mental equilibrium, are the best that can be hoped for?

3 ⌒

The Autonomic
Nervous System (ANS)

B efore approaching the physiological mechanisms that are set in motion by the organism's response to stress, it is best to be somewhat familiar with the primary driver of this adaptation: the Autonomic Nervous System (ANS). The ANS is a division of the peripheral nervous system that functions involuntarily and reflexively.

We shall attempt to present the organization and functioning of this system as clearly as possible, so the reader may glimpse a part of the beauty and magnificent precision that is our physical self. I think it is important not to be a stranger to our body and the extraordinary activity that unfolds continuously at its center. Nevertheless, the reader is certainly free to skip the details of this chapter and still be able to understand the rest of the book.

The ANS developed to serve an essential goal: the survival of the organism. Together with the hormonal and immune systems, it forms one of three pillars that permit continuous growth, regulation, balance, and stability. The ANS is responsible for constantly adapting the body to environmental changes, both internal and external, and is fast to react.

The autonomic nervous system allows us to survive dangerous situations by mobilizing us into sustained activity in an emergency. In the event we meet up with a lion, for example, the ANS prepares us for fight or flight through physiological responses that give us almost super human-like levels of strength and power to cope with the threat.

However, with the onset of illness, the ANS ceases to function optimally. Indeed, a dysfunctional ANS is a precursor to the manifestation of the vast majority of disease conditions. Because this system regulates our vital functions, without a highly functional ANS it becomes difficult to recuperate and recover good health. Furthermore, emotional and mental balance are central to a vibrant ANS. With this in mind, it is easy to understand the importance of cultivating personal equanimity. One is no longer astonished at the sheer number of individuals now in fragile health, not to mention the mounting financial and social cost that attends. It would seem that a great many human beings have difficulty managing their emotional make up, something at once fragile and so powerful, that it conditions our very existence.

The ANS automatically regulates:

- heart rate;
- respiration and the bronchi;
- body temperature;
- all digestive functions;
- metabolism;
- urinary functions; and
- sexual functions.

It also interacts with the hormonal and immune systems.

The ANS is made up of two opposing and complementary divisions: the sympathetic and parasympathetic. The para-sympathetic system is also known as the *vagal system,* deriving its name from the nerve that composes a great part of it. Every organ, tissue, and gland receives nerve endings from both divisions, except for blood vessels, which are almost entirely innervated by the sympathetic system. The sympathetic and parasympathetic systems operate somewhat like a break and an accelerator, for most of the organs. Sometimes, their action is a little more complex. To take the analogy of a steam locomotive, the action of the sympathetic system consists in adding coal to the boiler to provide fuel to power the train, while the role of the parasympathetic is to restock coal reserves once the train is stopped.

Functions of the sympathetic nervous system

The sympathetic system switches on as soon as the organism enters into action or work (ergotropic function). It stimulates all mechanisms responsible for mobilizing energy reserves for activity, such as the release of glucose, all with a purpose to increase blood levels in the brain, heart, and muscles at the expense of circulation to the organs and skin.

Functions of the parasympathetic system

This system is active during periods of rest and recuperation, and predominates in the night. It is responsible for the maintenance and repair of cells and tissues (trophotropic function), preserving energy and restoring depleted "nourishment" supplies. It is involved in certain pathological phenomena such as swooning or fainting (vagal episode), bowel diseases (colitis, for example), diarrhea, vomiting, tear production, and so forth. At rest, parasympathetic activity predominates in the heart and the smooth muscles of the digestive and urinary systems.

Autonomic tone

Tone refers to the level of activity level of the two nervous systems. Tone can be normal (normotonic), excessive (hypertonic), or insufficient (hypotonic).

In most stressed individuals, the sympathetic system is over stimulated. The resulting state of sympaticotonia underlies a great many symptoms, as we shall see in future pages. The term sympaticotonia is used when the sympathetic system is in overdrive, whereas vagotonia denotes parasympathetic dominance.

Sympathetic tone generally corresponds to the left cerebral hemisphere, while the parasympathetic system is linked with the right hemisphere. The two systems favor the states or modalities represented in Table 1.

TABLE 1

SYMPATHETIC	PARASYMPATHETIC
Activity	Receptivity
Speeding up	Slowing down
Tension	Relaxation
Focus	Global perspective
Convergent thoughts	Divergent thinking
Extraversion	Introversion
Goal oriented	Process oriented
Direction	Elaboration

The two divisions have complementary effects on organs and functions, as depicted in Table 2.

TABLE 2

ORGAN	SYMPATHETIC	PARASYMPATHETIC
Sweat glands	Stimulation	No effect
Hair	Goose bumps	No effect
Pupil	Dilation	Constriction
Lacrimal glands	No effect	Secretion
Heart	Acceleration	Slowing down
Coronary arteries	Dilation	No effect
Muscular arteries	Dilation	No effect
Cutaneous arteries and other arteries	Constriction	No effect
Bronchi	Dilation	Constriction
Bronchial secretions	Decreased	Stimulated

(continued)

ORGAN	SYMPATHETIC	PARASYMPATHETIC
Digestive system		
Secretions	Decreased	Stimulated
Peristalsis	Diminished	Accelerated
Rectum	Fills	Evacuates
Smooth sphincters	Contracted	Relaxed
Spleen	Contraction	No effect
Urinary system		
Secretions	Diminished	Augmented
Peristalsis	Diminishes	Increases
Bladder	Relaxes	Empties
Smooth sphincter	Contracts	Relaxes
Sex organs	Ejaculation/orgasm	Erection
Adrenal medulla	Secretion++	No effect
Metabolism	Catabolism	Anabolism

ANS Imbalances

The marvelous system that is the ANS can, for any number of reasons, become dysregulated. Given that base regulation must stay within certain limits, tone level varies among individuals. Some people are constitutionally more "sympathetic" and others more "parasympathetic" than average. Listed below are the main signs that one of the two systems is over stimulated or at least dominates the activity of the other.

Sympaticotonia (sympathetic) is marked by:

- drying of the eyes, sinuses, and mouth (diminished secretions);
- pupil dilation (mydriasis);
- arterial constriction, palpitations, and elevated blood pressure;

- localized sweating;
- slowed digestion (to reduce energy expenditure);
- loosening of the intestines;
- relaxation of the bladder;
- general stimulation of the entire organism;
- lowered immunity;
- irritability and insomnia;
- sexual signs/premature ejaculation; and
- all problems linked to an overextended period of the general adaptation syndrome response to stress.

Vagotonia (parasympathetic) is marked by:

- hypersecretions, general slowdown, and sometimes obesity;
- anxiety, depression, and hypersomnia;
- subject tends to be calm, timid, introverted, asthenic, with a depressive tendency, easily discouraged;
- skin: tendency towards greasiness, allergies, polyps, and dermatosis;
- general feebleness;
- tendency to be overweight;
- hypotension, syncope (temporary loss of consciousness through a drop in blood pressure) lipothymia, varicosities, migraine, and vertigo;
- aerophagia, gastritis, ulcers, diarrhea, nausea, vomiting, and intestinal spasms;
- spasmodic colitis, with alternating diarrhea and constipation;
- enuresis;
- sinusitis, rhinitis, asthma, chronic bronchitis and labored breathing;
- pain in the solar plexus; and
- impotence and vaginismus.

Brief anatomical description

The anatomy of the ANS is complex and can be a little daunting to the reader who is unfamiliar with the study of anatomy. Simply imagine command centers located in the brain, whose integrating and regulatory functions are activated by a network of cables linked to all parts of the body.

Brain centers

Three distinct brains emerged successively in the course of evolution, and now co-inhabit the human skull (Figure 1). While biological functions and behaviors have become increasingly elaborate, the human being carries within him the evolutionary strata of the animal kingdom, of which the triune brain model reminds us.

Each of the three brains performs functions related to the ANS.

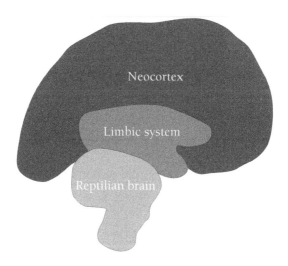

Figure 1. The three brains.

A. The reptilian brain

Our reptilian brain is more like the entire brain of modern day reptiles. It constitutes the deepest brain layer, and houses our archaic instincts. Structures include the brain stem (located at the base of your skull), hypothalamus, and the striatal complex. This ancient part of the brain is involved with reflexive instinctive behavior, territoriality, and the reproductive imperative. It is the center of survival of the self and the species.

Basic functions include:

- hormonal control;
- temperature control;
- respiration and heart beat;
- reproduction;
- fight or flight response; and
- hunger and thirst.

The striatum helps co-ordinate motivation with body movements, generating instinctual behavior characteristic of a species, such as posturing, aggression, submission, preening, and mating.

The hypothalamus is the true autonomic brain, linked to all other parts of the brain involved with the ANS. The hypothalamus governs general physiological functions, such as arterial tension and heart rate, regulates sleep cycles, and governs alimentary activity, as it contains the hunger and satiety centers. Reproduction and the hormonal cycle—more apparent in females—are also under its control. By way of its close relationship with the pituitary gland (involved in the production of many hormones), it orchestrates all endocrine glands, including the thyroid and adrenals. It plays a role in emotional self—regulation and motivation, together with the limbic system.

B. The paleomamallian brain or limbic system

The limbic system emerged in the first mammals. It is made up of many structures located at the inner surface of the cerebral hemispheres, and includes the part of the brain involved with smell, which is why it is also known as the rhinencephalon. This reflex apparatus influences the autonomic nervous system in response to emotional circumstances, and is the probable seat of psycho-visceral centers. Psychosomatic interaction means that emotions can engender physical disorders and illnesses.

The limbic system records the memory of behaviors that produced agreeable and disagreeable sensations, such as pleasure, desire, wrath, fear, joy, tenderness, and the like. It mediates our relationships, sense of belonging to a group, and the need to be recognized. This part of the brain is involved in homeostasis and equilibrium, and is thus intimately linked to the body.

Basic functions include:

- territorial management;
- fear;
- anger;
- aggression;
- maternal love;
- anxiety;
- hatred; and
- jealousy.

The limbic system includes structures such as the amygdala and the hippocampus that participate in the organism's stress response.

The amygdala is a paired mass of neurons that have an important role in coordinating aggressive behavior in response to fear. These neurons create a link between environmental stimuli and resulting behavioral responses. By evaluating the emotional value accorded events, the amygdala helps determine the nature of the stimulus and what the organism should do about it. Unfortunately, this part of the brain often generates conditioning connected to emotional learning, in which a neutral stimulus acquires aversive properties. It is thus that an individual can be conditioned to avoid fear-inducing stimuli or develop irrational phobias that can either restrain his activities or cause inappropriate defensive responses and aggressive behavior.

C. The neo-mammalian brain or neocortex

The neocortex sits atop the two preceding brain complexes, both anatomically and evolutionarily. This cerebral zone is particularly well developed in humans. It has two hemispheres. The left hemisphere enables our capacity for language, as well as analytical, linear, logical, and reasoned thought. The right hemisphere associates with intuition, creative, holistic, and spontaneous thought. The neocortex generates our capacity for adaptation and creativity, and is assumed to be responsible for the evolution of human intelligence.

Specific to our species is the prefrontal cortex, located behind the forehead. It is implicated in decision making, and gives us the ability to modulate thoughts and actions in accordance with internal goals. This part of the brain, characteristic of higher vertebrates, enabled the development of *homo sapiens* (man conscious of being conscious).

The neocortex provides judgement and discrimination, enabling the complex mental activities we associate with being human: the ability to think, imagine, reason, remember, learn, engage in logical and conceptual thought, forethought, and anticipation. The neocortex processes information coming from the whole body, as well as what reaches it from the outside world through the sense organs.

Cortical centers related to the ANS are not particularly well known or differentiated.

- The prefrontal zone and sub-orbital zones regulate the psyche—those characteristics of an individual that makes up his personality. It provides a neurophysiological link, where consciousness associates with the reticular formation and the hypothalamus. The prefrontal lobe plays an essential role in:

24

  - extraction, filtering, and analysis of significant information;
  - anticipation and selection of goal directed patterns of behavior; and
  - provisional memory, meaning the transient holding of new and task relevant information.
- The insular lobe is located within the cortical zones, between the frontal and temporal lobes; the insula play a role in diverse visceral and autonomic functions.
- Basic function of the neocortex includes:
  - anticipation;
  - fine perception;
  - differentiation between thoughts and feelings;
  - selection of appropriate behavior;
  - introspection and self-awareness;
  - elaborate approach to problems and solutions; and
  - goal fulfillment.

The autonomic pathways

In addition to the aforementioned cerebral centers, the ANS is mediated by nerves that emerge from the spinal cord, and relate to organs at specific spinal levels (see Figure 2). On exiting the spinal cord, sympathetic fibers distribute to organs and form nerve plexuses, such as the familiar solar plexus.

The parasympathetic neurons are located almost exclusively in the brain at the level of the brain stem, with some beginning at the inferior end of the spinal cord, the parasympathetic sacrum. Two especially important cranial nerves pass from the skull to the body. The right and left vagus nerves transport parasympathetic influx to most organs, and contribute parasympathetic fibers to the same nerve plexus formed by the sympathetic nerves. The pelvic organs (bladder, genital organs, end part of the colon) are dependent on the sacral parasympathetics.

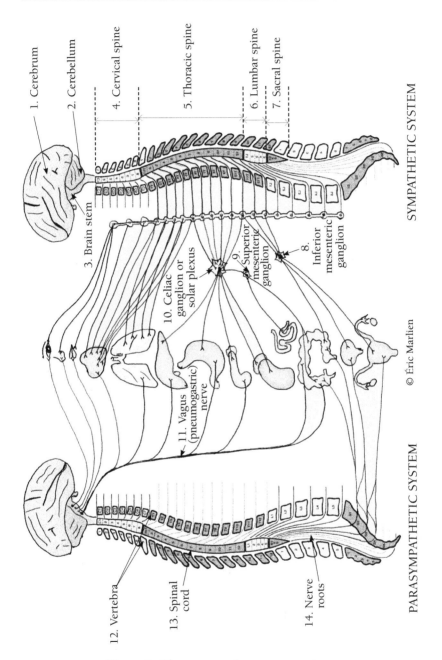

Figure 2. The autonomic nervous system.

1. Cerebrum
2. Cerebellum
3. Brain stem
4. Cervical spine
5. Thoracic spine
6. Lumbar spine
7. Sacral spine
8. Inferior mesenteric ganglion
9. Superior mesenteric ganglion
10. Celiac ganglion or solar plexus
11. Vagus (pneumogastric) nerve
12. Vertebra
13. Spinal cord
14. Nerve roots

SYMPATHETIC SYSTEM

PARASYMPATHETIC SYSTEM

© Éric Marlien

4 ⟋

The General Adaptation Syndrome

The General Adaptation Syndrome (GAS) represents a group of general physiological, neurological, endocrine, and immune mechanisms that regulate the organisms short-term and long-term reactions to stress. If, for example, you stay too long in the summertime sun, the symptoms of sunstroke are the manifestations of the GAS, while sunburn itself constitutes the specific reaction to the specific stressor, in this case a hot sun. The GAS represents a three-stage reaction to stress.

The stages of GAS

The alarm response

The alarm stage is the "fight or flight" response, first described by Walter Bradford Cannon. The immediate reaction to a perceived stress represents "the group of non-specifically generated phenomena provoked by the organism's sudden exposure to a harmful agent, a stimulus or stressor that the organism is not quantitatively or qualitatively adapted to."[1] It begins with the shock stage, when a cascade of adrenaline is discharged to create a boost of energy in the face of any brutal, violent, or intense situation. Such adrenaline flashes are so much sought today by the young—or the least young!

[1] Lôo Pierre, Lôo Henri et Galinowski André, *Le stress permanent*, Masson, 1999, p.6.

In the space of a few dozen milliseconds, the hypothalamus sends a general alarm out across the entire sympathetic nervous system and the body is rapidly awakened to action. Physiological changes instantaneously enable the body to combat stress in the most immediate way possible. Non-essential activities are reduced (digestive, urinary, and reproductive), while increased blood flow and energy are made available for rapid use by the heart, muscles, and brain.

This stage lasts anywhere from a few minutes to several hours. Assuming the individual survives, a counter-shock stage ensues, dominated by adrenocortical hormones. The circulation of glucocorticoids functions to increase gluconeogenesis, whereby sugar is produced from proteins and lipids that come from accumulated reserves in the body. This is in contrast to the initial stage, during which adrenaline draws on immediately available sugar reserves.

The resistance stage

If the stressful condition persists, the body adapts by a continued effort in resistance, and remains in a state of arousal (Figure 3). Depending on the intensity of the general adaptive response, outward signs of the first stage can either disappear or be accentuated. As the body continues to adapt, health can suffer because so much energy is concentrated on the reaction to stress, leaving it vulnerable.

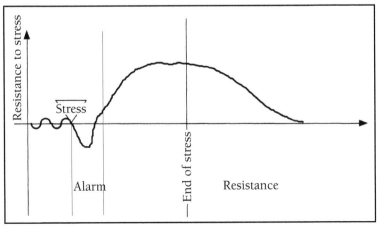

Figure 3. The resistance stage.

The exhaustion stage

The body enters into the exhaustion stage after stress has persisted for a long time, and the body's ability to resist is lost through the depletion of all physiological reserves (Figure 4). The signs of the alarm response reappear fleetingly, but the body's adaptive energy is gone and can no longer prevent the organism from succumbing to depression, burn out, serious illness, and even death.

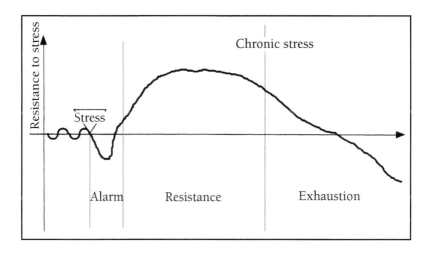

Figure 4. The exhaustion stage.

It can come as a surprise to people that this stage in the general adaptation system is so very hazardous to health.

Various effects of the exhaustion stage include:
- accelerated aging;
- brain cell death;
- bone density loss and increased osteoporosis;
- loss of muscle mass;
- reduced skin renewal and regeneration; and
- increased fat around the trunk, hips, face and neck.

Somatic pathologies include:
- hypertension;
- arteriosclerosis;
- myocardial infarction and other cardiovascular problems;
- constipation, colitis, and ulcer;
- diabetes;
- infertility;
- inflammatory responses;
- obesity;
- impaired immune function and immune deficiency disorders;
- cancer; and
- alzheimer's disease.

Psychic disorders include:
- indifference, introversion, diffidence, passivity, and resignation;
- depression;
- anorexia;
- anxiety; and
- impaired learning and memory.

Behavioral changes include:
- irritability; and
- increased risk of accident through carelessness and negligence.

Mechanisms of the GAS

Chronic stress can involve numerous functions of the nervous, autonomic, and endocrine systems. These are fully described in numerous books, and the reader who wishes to know more can easily reference them himself.[1]

---

[1] See for example, Lôo Pierre, Lôo Henri et Galinowski André, *Le stress permanent*, Masson, 1999. Millenson J.R., *Le corps et l'èsprit*, DésIris, 1998. Rossi E.L., *Psychologie de la guérison*, Le Souffle d'Or, 2002.

Science is increasingly aware of the effects of stress on the immune system and how it weakens, in almost all cases, resulting in sickness or disease. A simple familiar example is the common cold that frequently occurs following a period of stress, after exams in students, or during the first few days of vacation in overworked professionals.

Another component of the stress response shows up as changes in base muscle tone. Hypertonia affects all muscles, particularly those involved in standing and countering gravity, such as at the neck.

Prolonged hypertonia of muscle groups first causes painful tension, then joint movement limitation, followed by compression of joint surfaces, leading to biochemical changes to synovial fluid,[1] and finally, a wearing of cartilage surfaces and peri-articular structures. All of this is a complicated way of saying that arthritis eventually settles in.

A commonly observed example of this stress phenomenon is seen in the muscles of mastication; people with such a tendency often clench their teeth and grind them at night (bruxism), causing considerable dental wear. They complain of jaw pain and frequently wake up with neck pain. It is not far-fetched to imagine this tendency is of phylogenetic[2] origin. In many species, the function of the jaws, teeth, and supporting structures is directly linked with aggressive survival behavior—biting in order to defend or eat.

Global integration of the stress response

The body, via the brain, initiates the same biological response, whether the stressor is psycho-emotional or physiochemical in nature, save a few specific reactions involved in the latter. The following describes the body's integrated response to psycho-emotional stress (see Figure 5). The instant

---

[1] Synovial fluid nourishes and protects cartilage.
[2] Phylogenesis is the study of the formation, evolution, and genealogy of living beings.

a situation or event is perceived as stressful through the sensory organs, a complex set of direct influences and feedback actions are put into play, the full details of which we shall spare the reader. In any event, the way any particular stressor affects an individual depends on the factors listed below. While we are powerless, or relatively powerless over the two first parameters, the others are amenable to change, being open to our freedom of choice.

The first parameter is the very nature of a stressor can affect people differently. A mosquito bite or snakebite does not have the same impact on the body. The second parameter is the person's individual constitution can affect the way a person reacts to a stressor. A snakebite is more dangerous to a small child than to a robust man.

The third parameter is the value an individual ascribes to a particular stress depends on associations. The sight of a mouse can elicit mild interest, indifference, or outright terror and panic, depending on personal history. A given stressor may have caused a pleasant, unpleasant, or neutral response in the past or indeed be entirely unknown to a person. Familial, social, national, and cultural context all play into our reactions. In Figure 5, the recollection of a past traumatic session in the dentist leads to a wrong perception of the situation: the subject imagines that he will again definitely experience a painful situation and set in motion the mechanisms of stress. Results: increased orthosympathetic tone accentuates painful perceptions and the session will be traumatic, as the imagination predicted. The memorization of the painful state inherent in the dentist session is reinforced and the vicious circle is triggered.

The forth parameter is the level of perceived control in a person's ability to act or be forced to endure a situation. The neuro-endocrine axis mediates differently, depending on the case. When stress is within our control, mechanisms arise to either change or face up to and adapt to a situation. These responses are costly in terms of energy, and require a recuperation stage, at least as long as the adaptation stage. When stress overwhelms the emotional and mental resources of an individual, or when the situation is truly menacing, there are two possible responses.

The first response, which is rarer, is the sudden activation of the parasympathetic system, our most ancient autonomic branch. In the course of evolution, animals first adopted a strategy of passing out or playing dead in the face of a threat. When a person is unable to act in "fight or flight," the same primitive, if less effective, freeze response is deployed. The toned-down version of this reaction is called the vagal response, or syncope, a type of fainting linked to an overwhelming emotion. This is how a sensitive person, faced with a shock, can die of cardiac arrest.

The second response, which is more common, is the resistance stage, described above, which may lead to the exhaustion stage. The neocortex (frontal lobe in particular) loses control of the situation and the subject feels victimized, with no means of escape. The limbic system dominates (and the subject is dominated by his/her emotions), and through the intermediary of the hypothalamus and the hippocampus, activates the pituitary, corticosteroids, and many other systems.

The hippocampus is the territorial specialist and arbiter of social conventions. This part of the brain indexes long term memory, organizing and storing a person's worldview established through their experience. The Limbic-Hypothalamic-Pituitary-Adrenal Axis (LHPA) reveals the close relationship between a person's emotional life, which is underpinned by the limbic system and the pre-frontal cortex, and the neuroendocrine reaction to stress.

This axis sits at the interface between the subject's inner and outer worlds. It provides biological vigilance by controlling reactions to stress and regulating many body processes.

The hormonal response to stress signals the brain that the experience of defeat is so important on the biological plane that it must never be forgotten. Since conception, every experience is rated in terms of its potential impact on the survival of the individual or level of threat to physical and mental integrity.[1]

The hippocampus plays a determinant role in our lives, as it is one of the rare cerebral zones that can regenerate neurons from stem cells. The hippocampus is involved in consolidating memory, and this function can change in the course of life experiences.

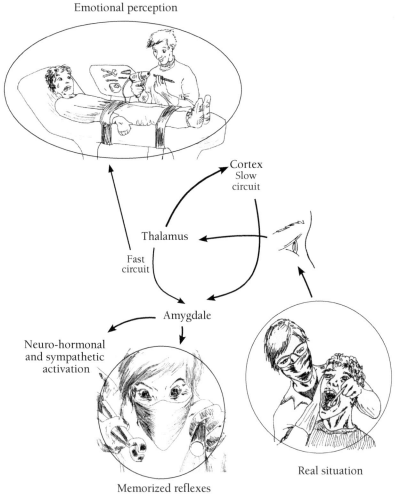

Figure 5. Birth of a psycho-emotional stress.

---

[1] Dantzer Robert, *L'Illusion psychosomatique*, Odile Jacob, 1989, p.75.

In summary, the more often an event repeats itself, bringing with it a cascade of physiological, emotional, and mental consequences, the more easily it can be reproduced, either negatively or positively. This system of reinforcement can drive a vicious or a virtuous cycle.

In addition, any thought or emotion belonging to this cycle can engender the exact same reactions. This is known as *memory linked to state,* where a pleasant or unpleasant memory is able to cause the same response, of more or less the same intensity, as the original experience. This is, of course, the story of Proust's precious madeleines whose very scent was enough to revive intense feelings and sensation from the author's boyhood.

It is entirely possible to break a vicious cycle in which we can find ourselves confined. We hope that the next chapters can help you to identify cycles in which you might find yourself stuck. Strange to say, but it is fairly common for us to be completely unaware that we are not well. "That's life" and "I am just like everyone else" are all expressions that mask our conditioning, and hinder our capacity to change.

5 ⌒⌐

Cardiac coherence

C ardiac coherence is a new approach to health based on the scientific analysis of a phenomenon called Heart Rate Variability (HRV). The study of HRV gives an excellent picture of the performance and adaptive flexibility of our autonomic nervous system, but also of our state of stress and our emotional balance. HRV is the subject of thousands of articles across the world.

Our emotional state influences the rhythm of the heart, and our heart rhythm also influences our brain. Neuroscience has demonstrated that the heart has its own "small brain" possessing an independent nervous system comprising as many as 40,000 neurons, all closely linked to the emotional brain. This amounts to a "heart-brain" system, explaining how the heart has considerable influence over our emotional states.

What we call cardiac coherence is a state in which our sympathetic and parasympathetic systems function in a coordinated and harmonious manner, ensuring adapting variations in our heart rate that influence all other major systems of the body. Whenever the heart functions in coherence, it secretes various hormones that stimulate the entire body and interact with the immune system. In this way, the heart acts as a powerful oscillator, able to bring all other systems of the body, and certainly the cerebrum, into a state of optimal function.

Essential concepts

Cardiac coherence is an expression of heartbeat variation under the influence of the sympathetic and parasympathetic branches of the ANS. These fluctuations take in to account two main parameters.

1. The physiological increase and decrease of the intervals between heart beats during the cardiac cycle (see arrows in Figure 6). The pulse regularly accelerates and decelerates, meaning its frequency is never stable. Whenever a heart is described as beating at 70 beats per minute, this figure displays the average heart rate. In the same way, if you take an hour to drive 100 kilometers, the car travels at an average speed of 100 km/h, but with stretches along the way ranging between 40 to 120 km/h. A perfectly regular heart is paradoxically a sign of serious illness. However, do not be alarmed if, in taking your pulse, it appears to be regular. The variations we are talking about here are difficult for the bare hand to perceive. If on the other hand, you should ever feel your physical heart beating irregularly, you are picking up arrhythmia (usually benign) but something that requires medical investigation nevertheless.

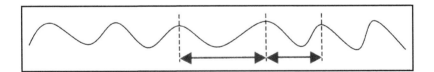

Figure 6.
Simple curve of six heart beats

2. The delta between strongest and weakest cardiac frequency (double arrows in Figure 7) registers when the subject is at rest and immobilized. Normally the rate rises on inhalation and falls on exhalation.

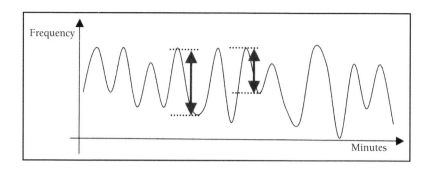

Figure 7.
Heart rate wave.

The wave in Figure 7 is not to be confused with the wave depicted in Figure 6. The curve above registers waves over two minutes, or about 140 heartbeats. It represents the frequency in the course of 10 slow and deep inhalations. This would represent the recording of the instantaneous speed along a route, while the curve of figure 6 would represent each turn of the wheel. Example: during one inspiration, the frequency rate increases by 6 or 7 beats, then diminishes on exhalation over the course of 7 other beats. We have a recording, whose oscillations reflect respiratory cycles, during which many heartbeats occur.

The relationship between these two parameters is reflected by a key indicator called Heart Rate Variability (HRV), improperly called cardiac coherence in extensive articles. Cardiac coherence describes a state in which the brain's activities are synchronized with those of the heart, resulting in a physiological state of well-being.

Breathing influences the way the ANS regulates heart rate. Inhalation inhibits the influence of the parasympathetic system (loosening of the vagal brake) and increases heart rate, while exhalation stimulates the parasympathetic system and decreases heart rate.

Heart rate variability can appear on a graph in two forms (see illustrations on pages 44, 46 and 48):

- chaotic (random, disordered) when we are under the influence of stress, anxiety, fear, or anger; and
- coherent (ordered) when we feel positive emotions, compassion, a state of wellbeing, or experience fond memories.

Good cardiac coherence is reflected in instantaneous variation in heart rate in relation to respiration, with a delta occurring between the maximal and minimal frequency. Inversely, poor cardiac coherence shows up as waves that are more or less chaotic, depending on the underlying imbalance. We shall see several examples in the graphs on the next few pages.

Cardiac variability reflects the physiological elasticity of the heart, as well as an optimally functioning ANS.

It reveals our emotional state, our capacity to organize information, make a decision, and resolve problems. It is above all an indicator of our flexibility and resiliency in terms of our environment and our ability to handle stress. Strong coherence is one of the best indicators of good health and well-being for all ages in both men and women.

Recent discoveries by the American University scientist Stephen W. Porges[2] show that the parasympathetic system is in fact a double system.

- The ancient part controls the abdominal organs, and is responsible for inhibitory mechanisms and the syncope described earlier.
- Another more recently evolved part mainly controls the heart and lungs.
  - This division of the parasympathetic system has been called the "social engagement system," because it is fully functional when a person is in a secure

[2] The polyvagal theory: phylogenetic substrates of a social nervous system. Stephen W. Porges. International Journal of Psychophysiology 42 Ž2001. 123 146

environment and engaged in rich and fulfilling social relationships.

– In this context, it slows down the heart rhythm, and its effectiveness is precisely what is measured by heart rate variability.

– This part of the nervous system allows us to modulate and mitigate the sympathetic responses to stress that are so costly to health. Research reveals its dominant role in maintaining optimal physical and mental health, as well as immunity.

Optimal cardiac coherence increases physical and intellectual capacities. Low cardiac coherence is a predictor of health problems. The combination of stress, poor diet, and sedentary lifestyle is responsible for the majority of diseases in the industrialized world, and is the cause of infinitely more deaths than those caused by war and terrorism. So, we see that which we should be concerned about.

The most easily measured indicators of weakened health are:

- high blood pressure;
- heightened cortisol levels;
- elevated glucose;
- elevated free fatty acids;
- elevated insulin;
- decrease in the size the left ventricle of the heart; and
- finally, a lowering of the heart rate variable, which shows up as a predictor of deteriorating health status well before other biological markers.

Although still to be taken under advisement, some American studies demonstrate that a person with good heart variability is much less likely to have a morbid prognosis, even when other markers are above normal. By contrast, favorable biological markers, when associated with lowered cardiac variability, are not in themselves guarantors of good health.

Pathways to harmonious cardiac coherence include the following:

- activities involving the body and mind (meditation,[3] yoga, psychotherapy, positive outlook on life—any means to understand how mental states affect behavior);
- functional modalities (movement therapy, osteopathy, sports, breathing, relaxation—any activity that improves the psychomotor relationship);
- cellular support (natural medications, nutrition, etc.).

This book outlines strategies pertaining to the first two pathways.

Cardiac coherence applications

- Improved management of:
  - stress and anxiety;
  - negative emotions; and
  - pain.

- Overcoming:
  - obesity;
  - depression; and
  - addiction.

- Preventing:
  - cardiovascular disease;
  - mood disorders; and
  - preserving optimal health.

- Improving:
  - psychological health; and
  - athletic performance.

---

[3] Meditation is likely the best way to improve our cardiac coherence.

- Other scientifically validated benefits include:
  - increased longevity;
  - fewer morbid thoughts;
  - greater cognitive flexibility;
  - improved memory;
  - better decision making;
  - heightened creativity and innovation in problem solving; and
  - enhanced work performance.

Measuring cardiac coherence

The heart's rhythm can be easily measured and graphed by specialized software program (described below) and an ear clip sensor or fingertip device that is linked to a monitor connected to a computer. But the best systems are those that do the analysis according to an electrocardiogram. The analysis of the data gathered by this feedback device, is best done at least for the first time, is best done by a competent and experienced person. Despite assertions made by the companies that market the software, data interpretation is not entirely simple and can lead to erroneous findings.

Examples of cardiac coherence graphs

Nowadays several companies market software that measures cardiac variability. The most advanced system for obtaining as much data as possible, including an accurate evaluation of each part of the autonomic nervous system, sympathetic and parasympathetic, is provided by the French company Codesna and its device Physioner©.

The following pages include cardiac coherence graphs by Codesna.

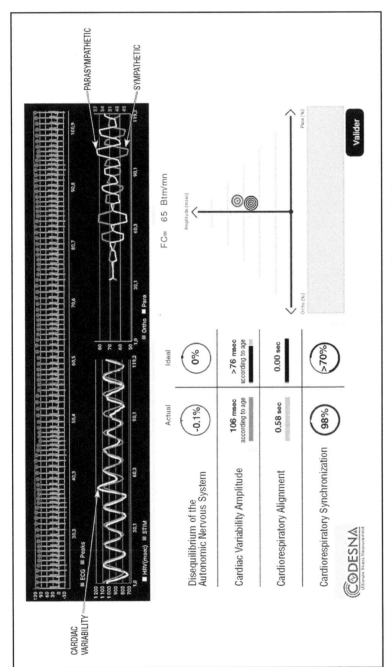

Figure 8. Subject calm and at ease with excellent ANS balance.

Subject calm and at ease with excellent ANS balance (Figure 8)

Equilibrium is almost perfect. The target is almost centered, barely offset from the parasympathetic side. The cardiac variability is a quasi-sinusoid with an amplitude greater than average (meaning a powerful ANS). The perceived stress questionnaire also revealed a very good emotional balance.

The sympathetic and parasympathetic curves show a good alternation and a perfect synchronization between the two systems in relation to breathing.

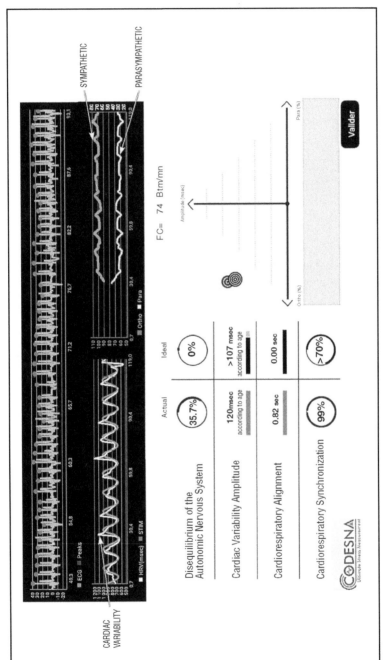

Figure 9. The subject is stressed with sympathetic system predominant.

Subject stressed with predominant sympathetic system (Figure 9)

The sympathetic system is dominant (35.7%), which reflects a state of stress. The target is shifted on the sympathetic side. The sympathetic curve is stronger than the parasympathetic curve, reflecting a sympathetic tone stronger than the parasympathetic tone. The cardiac variability amplitude remains still powerful (120 msec) compared to the average for his age (107 msec), meaning adaptation possibilities still preserved for the moment. Over time, there is a risk of decompensation from exhaustion. The stress perception questionnaire revealed both a professional and a personal problem. Such a subject will very likely end up exhausted and serious pathologies may turn up.

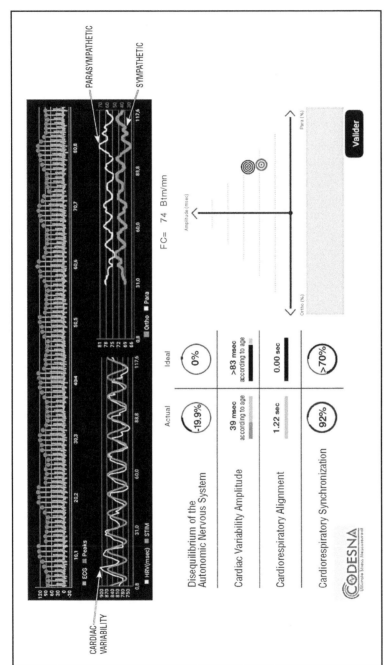

Figure 10. Subject in vagotonia, parasympathetic system predominant.

Subject in vagotonia with predominant parasympathetic system (Figure 10)

When there is an important parasympathetic tone dominant (19.9%), the curve is higher than the sympathetic one and the target is shifted on the parasympathetic side. The small cardiac variability amplitude (39 msec) is compared to the average for its age (83 msec). This may be due to certain temporary forms of fatigue or beta-blocking drugs. Stress is generally not present in this type of patient. Depressive states can also give this type of measure.

Conclusion

There are, of course, many other types of recordings, and the system developed by the company Codesna allows a much more precise clinical analysis of the ANS and the consequences of stress on our health. From a certain age, often as early as 30 years, it is more common to observe states of disturbance rather than a balanced ANS. Stress and emotional imbalances are actually the number one public enemy.

Alas, many among us have gone through an existential crisis or maelstroms of anxiety and overwork. It is important to be aware that these factors weigh heavily on our health, and these graphs can be a good warning of what can happen.

Modern medicine appears to underestimate the impact of stress and emotional imbalances. Media advertisers persuade people into giving over responsibility for their well-being to government and medical authorities, whose response is sometimes to enlist the goodwill of large pharmaceutical companies.

If it is of course absurd to question the excellent medical research performed in the realm of public health. However, it a shame not to see the same level of study devoted to understanding individuals in possession of good physical and psychological health in an attempt to understand the factors that guarantee and support wellbeing.

Prevention, through such understanding, is the greatest of all medicine. The study of cardiac coherence is truly part of this future.

PART TWO

Ways and Means
in Practice

Practical Work

⌒

W hat follows are practical ways for you to change profoundly, albeit gradually, your physiological, mental, and emotional balance. The goal is to see that changes in the way you live can help you better manage stress and, by living more positively, develop honest and equitable relationship with yourself and others. Needless to say, this may not happen overnight! Time and consistency are required to transform habits of being that are often longstanding, having become entrenched over the years.

This is why the practical work which follows is constructed according to an important progression, which needs to be respected. We have divided this work into phases—one for each level—physiological, emotional, and mental. These are the three aspects that make up our human personality. In each section, you will find ideas to help you understand the causes and consequences of the problem reflected. Exercises and suggestions follow a coherent course. In general, each exercise must be experienced a number of times before moving on to the next. Lasting results are built on a sure foundation. "Make haste slowly." I suggest you do a preliminary read through of this chapter, trying your hand at the first two exercises.

The exercises in this first section are not necessarily to be undertaken in the precise order they appear. The arbitrary division of chapters into "physiological," "emotional," and "mental" is only meant to facilitate understanding, and provide some logic to the presentation. Their partition does not fully account for their interrelationships.

One cannot very easily find emotional calm and serenity in an ill-at-ease and tension-filled body. Accordingly, the program sometimes draws exercises from different sections, with a view to overall physiological, emotional, and mental balance.

A "calendar" and observation chart are provided in the endnotes. Week by week you will be shown the steps required and number of days suggested for their practice as you progress level by level. This schedule is only a suggestion, and can be adapted according to your needs or inclination. With genuine desire and steady determination, it is likely that in a matter of weeks you, as well as those around you, will notice real and profound change.

1 〜

Attaining cardiac coherence: physiological equilibrium

Breathing

The main function of respiration is, of course, to provide gaseous exchange between blood and air: the intake of oxygen and giving off of carbon dioxide. Shallow breathing diminishes blood oxygen levels and reduces vitality available to all cells that depend on oxygen for their metabolic activity. Every cell in the organism carries out a specific function, depending on the organ or tissue to which it belongs.

Brain neurons have the greatest oxygen requirement of all body cells. A brain deprived of oxygen cannot perform optimally. Thoughts are less clear; intelligence goes down; decision making suffers; and the impact of negative emotions on the body is more pronounced. Reduced respiration also raises carbon dioxide levels in the blood. The resulting lowered blood pH is responsible for acidification of the body, one of whose consequences is increased muscle tension.

High quality respiration provides other important functions. Full and easy breathing is initiated by the diaphragm, our primary muscle of inspiration (Figure 13). The diaphragm has the shape of a dome, separating the thoracic cavity from the abdominal cavity (Figure 14). Accessory muscles of respiration support thoracic elevation, useful whenever the demand for oxygen increases significantly, such as during sports.

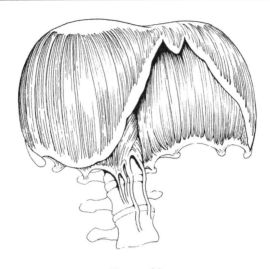

Figure 13.
The diaphragm (after Calais-Germain B.,
Respiration anatomie–geste respiratoire, Déslris, 2005, p.80).

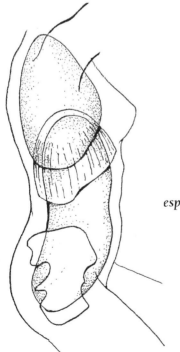

Figure 14.
Location of diaphragm
(after Calais-Germain B.,
espiration anatomie–geste respiratoire,
Déslris, 2005, p.86).

Under normal conditions, the thoracic cage is only moderately involved in breathing. When the diaphragm contracts, it moves downward during inspiration, and then passively moves upward during expiration. This rhythmic activity occurs over 20,000 times a day, providing a perpetual massage to the heart, as well as all abdominal organs. Intra-abdominal pressures fluctuate constantly, contributing to the optimal function of the digestive organs, as well as the circulatory, urogenital, and lymphatic systems.

Strong digestion and efficient transit depend on adequate diaphragm activity. Deep full breaths stimulate the venous and lymphatic systems, avoiding stasis in the abdomen and lower limbs. The superior drainage of the digestive organs, whose venous blood passes through the liver before returning to the heart, is critically important. The liver cleanses waste products from the organs and also metabolizes numerous elements essential to our health.

It is good to understand how the components of a vicious circle can be linked: stress, anxiety, and negative emotions can all limit respiration and engender muscle tension. The accompanying acidification and loss of organ stimulation, combined with reduced circulation, can cause all manner of disagreeable and painful conditions and tension. Such a state of malaise leaves us even more sensitive to stress and anxiety, which can lead to excessive emotional responses.

Breath education, or re-education, is one of the most effective techniques in revitalizing all levels of being. Apart from breaking a downward spiral, proper breathing generates a positive inner state and inspires us to feel or discover aspects of ourselves that we either never knew or have long since forgotten.

Guided breathing sets in motion a process of subtle and powerful change. This has been observed for ages by various Asian disciplines and philosophies. In traditions, such as yoga, spiritual practices/techniques found in Zen or Tibetan Buddhism, or the energy arts of Taoism—this is not by any means an exhaustive list—all begin with the breath.

Much can be learned from these ancient disciplines. In modern culture, life can appear somewhat denatured and certainly pressure-filled. Today's society is geared to push us outside ourselves in action, sensation, and emotions. The "stronger" these are, the more they are valued. It is not a question of adopting Asian cultural ways that have, of course, their own limitations, but to perhaps incorporate some features that have been given short shifts in our culture. Conscious breathing leads you to discover the richness of our inner vibration. This treasure can be valuable to ourselves, and opens up the outer world of our friends, work, and relationships.

In the practice of breathing, it is normal, at the beginning, to feel some tightness under the ribcage or at the solar plexus. If your breathing has been restricted for some time, or if you are in the habit of holding tension here, muscle and tendon fibers of the diaphragm must first be softened. So too must the peritoneum, the connective tissue that lines and surrounds organs, such as the stomach and liver. After a few days, fifteen at most, any discomfort will disappear and give way to a pleasant feeling and a level of ease you might not have even imagined at the outset.

If, however, you continue to experience pain or discomfort, it may be beneficial to consult an osteopath or a manual therapist. This will free the mobility restrictions of some of your joints, or of your thoracic and abdominal organs. This will allow you to regain the mobility of your tissues, and thus, ample and free breathing.

If you wish to keep track of your impressions, or any difficulties that might arise during the weeks, you can keep notes in the back of this book in the Observations and Progress section. This can be useful to track your progress towards new found balance.

Exercise 1: Observation

The first thing to do is simply notice your breath. As you read these lines and, without trying to control the rhythm, observe how your breath unfolds, identifying inspiration and expiration, and perceiving any differences that might exist between these two phases. Do you breathe in and out with equal ease? Which parts of the cycle seem more mobile? Does your belly inflate as your chest expands? Do you breathe through your nose, mouth, or both at once? Is your mouth open or closed? Is your respiration deep or shallow?

Close your eyes and place your attention on these questions for two or three minutes. At the end of the exercise, ask yourself if you succeeded in remaining focused on your breath, or did your thoughts have a tendency to disperse, follow their own path, or wander towards some current preoccupation? The answer to this question is already an indication of your ability to concentrate.

Practicing cardiac coherence

As I sit at my computer starting to write this chapter, I find myself having a hard time concentrating. I don't quite know how to begin. I remain distracted by the incessant comings and goings of my three-and-a-half-year-old son, who is playing in my study. Whereas, when I am able to concentrate, I can be quite indifferent to external agitation. This is just one example of many, where the practice of cardiac coherence can make a difference. I practice the exercise that follows for two or three minutes, in combination with a relaxed attitude and mental receptivity. And voila! as if by magic, the phrases that I am about to write come to the surface of my mind, without effort and the rest flows by itself.

Important preliminary remarks

The following advice applies, with a few exceptions, to all the exercises in this book. These rules will become second nature.

- Sit in a chair, spine erect. This posture works best for at least three reasons.
  - A slumped position does not permit the diaphragm to function correctly.
  - Posture reflects our interior attitude. The inverse is also true—posture influences our state of mind. Assume the posture of an ill at ease, rather apathetic adolescent, and you will easily feel how this works.
  - Spinal nerves emerge from our spinal column and distribute to all parts of the body. Good posture favors the unimpeded circulation of nerve impulses, which pass in two directions through these spinal segments.

Nevertheless, it is necessary that you be relaxed and not at all uncomfortable. Make use of a cushion to support the lumbar spine, if you like. Your head should not be held back. It should sit in line with the spine, or slightly forward. Avoid tight belts that limit the free expansion of your belly in inspiration. Make sure that your shoulders are at ease. The same goes for your jaw. Nervous people sometimes unwittingly clench their jaw. Place your feet flat on the floor. If you practice yoga and are accustomed to sitting cross-legged with your back straight without discomfort, you are welcome to adopt this position.

Finding a suitable breathing rhythm depends on several factors, such as your age, sex, weight, athletic ability, medical history, and more. Begin by slowing down your present rhythm a bit, without too much effort. Let a sense of ease and pleasantness be your guide. Find your breath becoming slower, fuller, and more even. Resting rhythm is about 15 cycles per minute, on average. Time your breath without any further attempt to slow it down. The goal is to reduce your starting rhythm by thirds, eventually achieving a rate of 5 to 6 cycles per minute, on average, after completing the relaxation exercises.

Allow the air to pass gently from the nostrils to the nasopharynx, the posterior part of the nasal cavity that joins the back of the throat. Forcing the breath risks inflaming the delicate mucosa that lines these parts, as well as overstimulating the brain. Hyperventilation is to be avoided also, as it can promote respiratory alkalosis of the blood, leading to dizziness, light-headedness, and in severe cases, tetany. Some psycho-therapeutic techniques are based on rapid breathing, but this is not at all the direction intended here.

Your breathing must always be nasal, lips closed, and teeth unclenched. Mouth breathing, beyond a certain age in childhood, is not a good thing.

Days in which you have a cold with a nose are best considered vacation days in breathing practice!

Exercise 2: Respiratory coherence

The objective here, aside from familiarizing yourself with conscious respiration, is to enter a state of cardiac coherence. Find a comfortable posture for meditation, as described above. Close your eyes and check that your body is relaxed. Breath evenly through the nose. During inspiration, first let your belly gently fill, and only then allow the chest rise, but not too much. During the expiration, follow the air passively, flowing out of your lungs, through your nose, in the reverse order, like deflating bellows: first the chest empties, then the belly. To help you initially perceive and control the smooth running of things, you can place one hand on your belly, and the other on your chest.

Begin by doing this exercise for 5 minutes. Gradually increase it to 10 minutes. If you were to see the recording of your cardiac activity, with the help of cardiac coherence analysis software, you would see that, as a rule, your coherence level rises in less than two minutes. With training, your coherence will rise more quickly.

For the rest of this book, we refer to this practice as *coherent respiration*. Other parameters will be added along the way, so that little by little you will build within yourself an automatic breathing pattern, one you can adopt easily and practice frequently.

Exercise 3: Physiological coherence

The goal of this exercise is to optimize the effect of cardiac coherence through the use of a primary motor function found in infants—grasping and suction. This technique can be useful in case of fatigue, or to prepare for any activity that requires lots of energy, such as athletic endeavor. In people who have difficulty concentrating, this breathing exercise will help them to keep their focus better.

The fundamentals are the same as for the *coherent respiration,* with these additions.

- During inhalation, tighten your jaw, stick your tongue to the roof of the mouth, and gradually clench your fists.
- During exhalation, slowly unclench your jaw, relax your tongue, and fully open your hands.

Be careful to coordinate your movements in time with the breathing cycles for the duration of the exercise, about 5 minutes.

Exercise 4: Heart coherence

While the vital importance of the physical heart is obvious, the heart is also an energetic center, and an important seat of human consciousness. For many of us, the solar plexus is our emotional center, which can become tense and even painful as soon our emotions threaten to overwhelm us or stress mounts up. Moreover, modern culture is very invested in things cerebral, and we commonly focus our attention on our brain. There is no need to abandon this characteristic, but it can be beneficial to expand our awareness and broaden our responsive capacities.

Focusing our attention at the heart center disengages us from negative emotions that pass through the solar plexus with all their psychosomatic consequences. This allows us to elevate and refine our emotions, and develop the intelligence of the heart. Heart and intelligence are not contradictory terms. Certain traditions describe an energy called love wisdom. Neuroscience has begun looking in the same direction, and demonstrated that emotional experiences are part of normal cognitive processes and reasoning.[1] Studying the presence of neurons in the heart shows that the organ has a direct influence on the brain.

One way to discover heart intelligence is by consistently practicing *coherent respiration,* with your attention centered on the heart region. At the beginning, you may find it easier to place your focus on the middle of your chest. With time, you will benefit from centering your mind a little deeper in the chest, nearer the vertebral column, between the shoulder blades.

For this new exercise, enter into *coherent respiration,* as described above. During inhalation, visualize the incoming air like a luminous energy, white or golden, that accumulates in the region of the heart. During exhalation, imagine this lustrous energy spreading throughout your entire body. Continue this for 5 to 10 minutes.

A variation involves releasing all tensions, encumbering thoughts, and burdensome worries by visualizing them as large amounts of smoke or grey dust leaving your nostrils. More and more brightness accumulates within, as grayness dissipates with each out breath. This practice will allow you to rediscover calmness and serenity quickly, whenever you wish. You will find yourself less easily overtaken by negative states.

Why is it that so many people who have a favorable experience with this type of practice find themselves unable to continue with it in the face of an especially difficult situation? The answer could be simply that they do not think of it when

---

[1] Damasio, Antonio, *Descartes' Error*, Odile Jacob, 1995.

they need it most. In other cases, a childish attitude is at play. There can be a certain satisfaction in enclosing oneself in a state of negativity, whether it be anger, nervousness, guilt, sulkiness, or sadness, which, if examined honestly, is often a form of self-pity. It is a clumsy way of releasing pent up feelings that we have no other way of working out. Expressing our inner negativity also broadcasts to people around us how we feel. Perhaps it is a way of demanding attention and seeking help that we find difficult to ask for directly.

The remedy is to decide that you have the inner resources to move forward positively. Make the decision that you will not be dominated by external situations or interior reactions. Decide to make affirmative changes in your life, beginning by deciding on the practice of coherence.

Some may say that this is easier said than done. But is there really an alternative? To get anywhere, it is necessary to begin by putting one foot out. Talking about sore feet while standing on hot coals is not the best option. Is it not smarter simply to just decide to go ahead and move?

While practicing the exercise in the midst of some emotional or mental difficulty, your thoughts might well divert your focus. Simply bring your attention back "within" to your breath and heart, as many times as it takes without blaming yourself. Every relapse overcome is a victory won, and an experience of self-mastery gained. Sooner or later you will be able to look back on the progress you have made towards building your powers of mindful concentration.

Know that it is possible, even recommended, to practice this coherence exercise with your eyes open, in public, anytime you feel the need. People around you will have no notion of what you are doing, and in a matter of two or three minutes, less with training, you will have regained your equanimity and composure.

As a final note, you can practice this basic exercise your entire life, as long as it appeals to you and you feel its fundamental benefits. The exercises that follow include variations you can add to deepen the experience. In time, you will no longer need to think about your breath when you sit for your practice. Through shear habit, you will have established a natural rhythm that belongs to you.

Breathing: going deeper

Over and above key physiological functions, full and easy breathing serves to produce other much subtler energetic effects. The Asian traditions have accumulated a significant and well codified body of knowledge on the energetic counterpart of our physical body. Western science, so long at odds with these millennia-year-old traditions, has begun little by little to delve into the more esoteric aspect of the human being,[1] whether it be the Chi of Traditional Chinese Medicine or the Prana that nourishes our etheric body in the Indo-Tibetan tradition.

Through conscious breathing, our energetic body vibrates to a particular rhythm, by which we are connected to a primordial pulsation. All the rhythms of our body derive from this fundamental impulse. It is part of the rhythms of nature, of which we are a part, and belongs, perhaps also, to the rhythms of the universe beyond.

Healthful eating and regular exercise are essential to good health, but are not in themselves sufficient. The regular practice of free and ample breathing is the best way to improve our vitality, for breath combines both energetic and physical effects.

Vibration is the subtle aspect of breathing we take in as Prana, the life force that circulates through our entire body. With a little practice, you can experience this energetic dimension that builds vitality. You may find that you sleep better, or require less sleep, giving you more time to go about your daily obligations, and to enjoy fulfilling activities.

---

[1] Recommended reading on this subject, is the work of James L. Oschman, "Energy medicine, the scientific basis." Churchill Livingston, 2000.

By force of habit, we are almost always doing something or other: working, thinking, talking. We end up believing that life comes *down to doing*. We can be quite unaware that in order to simply exist, thousands of complex processes constantly animate our body; biochemical, metabolic, and electrical operations carry on. These activities follow laws of rhythm and unfold in a cyclical manner. Our life and our health have everything to gain by harmonizing to the same rhythms that dictate phases of activity and rest, as well as spells of extraversion and introversion. In stopping periodically from "doing," and dedicating a little time to inner silence and conscious breathing, we can transcend our individuality and connect to the animating rhythm of life.

Exercise 5: Observation

Now that you have some experience with breath, through practicing the cardiac coherence exercises, return to passively observing your breath, as first instructed. What differences do you notice, if any, from the initial experience? If you have jotted down your first impressions, it will be easy to see your headway.

Continue to observe your rhythmic breath for 5 to 10 minutes with your eyes closed. It might be that you come across unusual feelings or thoughts, impressions that are a little bit out of the ordinary. It is enough to simply appreciate such encounters, with no need of explanation. The idea is to get a taste of vibrations within.

Exercise 6: Interlude and sound

It is now possible to refine your mastery of breathing. This time, practice *coherent breathing* concentrating on the transition between inhalation and exhalation, and then the changeover between exhalation and inhalation. Pay attention to this fleeting moment, without looking to lengthen it. Just be aware that the space between breaths is a moment in which time is suspended. A tiny moment of deep stillness and pure awareness—that is part of our being.

Do not be discouraged if, at first, you experience nothing much in this interlude. Each of us has our own rhythm and facility in certain realms, and resistance in others. This is not important. What matters is that you continue to practice. Benefits will inevitably manifest over time.

In yoga, it is said that the breath has its own sound. Inspiration carries the sound *so;* expiration carries the sound *hum.* This is the *so-hum* or *saha-hum,* which means "this I am." Listen to the sound of your own breath, and little by little you will tame the experience of "being."

Exercise 7: Pause at inhalation

Continue breathing *in coherence,* focusing your awareness on your heart center. Follow several rounds of inhalation and exhalation, becoming aware of the paradox of being both the one who directs the breath and the *being* who breathes you from within.

The next step is to pause your breath between inspiration and expiration. Increase the interval slowly. Take your time. Begin by stopping for just a second or two. Then each day, increase the time between breaths by two to three seconds. Do not pause for more than 15 seconds. This duration can be attained over a period of 8 to 15 days, provided you practice daily. It is up to you to perceive the motif—the exact moment—to catch your breath. The impulse is not only due to an oxygen debt. It is up to you to find your own answer. Know only that it has to do with *desire.*

Exercise 8: Pause at exhalation

This exercise is the same as exercise 7, except this time, the breath is suspended at the end of exhalation. As in the first exercise, take your time by extending the intervals very gradually over a period of days. However, this time, do not exceed 10 seconds. At the end of expiration, the need for oxygen occurs more suddenly, and the perception of the underlying desire, or wish, is less easily perceived than during the inhalation pause.

Complete this breathing practice according to the calendar set out in the endnotes. It is not a matter of continuously intentionally breathing continuously with these pauses during each round. Rather, the purpose is to allow you to experience certain states of awareness that come up in the gap between breaths.

After a set period of practice, a slight natural interlude will occur naturally with each breath, more qualitatively than quantitatively. That being said, nothing prevents you from revisiting these exercises, if you find them valuable.

A breathing rhythm that you will be able to achieve spontaneously is a very slow exhalation, ending very gradually, and at least twice as long as inspiration.

Breathing this way has the ability to strengthen the parasympathetic system, to further increase cardiac coherence, and to reduce anxiety attacks and the level of stress. A lot of profit, isn't it?

2

Emotional equilibrium

Many of us suffer from emotional imbalance of one kind or another, showing up as anything from a variety of physical problems to mental agitation, indecisiveness, perhaps apathy, and eventually an absence of peace and contentment. Emotions, when they are refined and elevated, are a source of joy and sublime states of consciousness. They also motivate many of our actions.

Problems begin when negative emotions take hold of us. Anger without the desire to improve, fear without common sense, shame or embarrassment without the desire to move forward are sterile emotions that harm us and, often time, others.

How can we manage our emotions and gradually elevate the nature of emotions that inhabit us? Ideally, we would never find ourselves having to deal with being emotionally overwhelmed. Does this seem impossible? Whatever your belief, or you believe, inevitably determines the answer. Our potential for change is far greater than conventional wisdom leads many of us to believe.

Emotional balance can seem difficult to come by, especially if our temperament tends towards impulsivity, or has been emotionally driven over a long period of time. Conscious breathing, practiced over sufficient time, can lead to far-reaching and enduring change. Keep in mind that emotional balance is only attainable in concert with physical and mental harmony. Many of us live in an "emotional body" that is saturated with clutter. The royal treatment might well be called the "elimination method," by which the goal is to rid ourselves gradually of harmful, unnecessary, and cumbersome emotions. In other words, to render the "emotional body" as crystal clear as possible, and allow it to be receptive to the best, truest, and most harmonious impressions and vibrations that human beings have the privilege in which to share.

The exercises in this chapter may help you come to terms with difficult, or even violent emotions, through a better understanding of their origins. The first step is to develop our potential for concentration and visualization. Breathing exercises certainly contribute to improved attentiveness. The other practices laid out in this book will serve to reinforce our abilities. Concentration and visualization are indispensable to bringing new things into our life. Nothing comes into our existence that has not first been formed as a mental image or concept. This is creative imagination.

The following exercise is designed to determine what type of sensory perception you respond to best, and to develop your capacity for visualization.

The term *visualization* usually evokes the formation of visual images in our mind's eye, our spirit. However, vision is only one of our five senses. While it may be many people's dominant sense, a fair share of the population has refined audition, and a third group is highly "kinesthetic," adept at the sense perception of movement. Taste and smell are other sensory modalities, employed to varying degrees, generally as secondary means of perception.

Many people say they are unable to visualize. The explanation is that typically they are forcing themselves to create mental images. It is better to begin imagining sounds or motor images, and with time, allow visual images to appear on the mental screen.

For some people, images tend to appear quite out of the blue—daydreams and fantasies, for example. However, these same people often find themselves unable to visualize at will. The solution lies in training. Progress, no matter what the endeavor, is achievable with perseverance.

Exercise 9: Visualization

You can choose to practice each phase of this exercise with your eyes open or closed.

1. *"Visual" visualization*

- Quietly bring to mind the image of a classroom blackboard or a white wall. Then see the number 6 in the middle. (If need be, imagine drawing the figure with chalk on the board or a paintbrush on the wall.) Next, conjure up a mental picture of the number 1, placing it to the right of the number 6, giving you the number 61. Add the number 7, making 617. Continue adding figures in this way, for as long as you can remember the total.

- Make a note of the number of figures you succeeded in visualizing. Score yourself from 1 to 10 as a measure of your ability, taking into account both the sum of numbers and the sharpness of the image.

- Next, visualize a splash of red in any form you like. Retain this image for ten or so seconds. Do the same with the colors orange, yellow, green, blue, and violet. Score this visualization on a scale of 1 to 10.

- Now imagine the face of one of your friends or family: the general appearance, shape, expression, including details such as eyes, nose, mouth, and so on. Evaluate the quality of what you see on a scale of 1 to 10.

- Then, visualize a series of geometric shapes, and hold each one in your mind's eye for several seconds: a point, circle, triangle, square, six-point star, a cube, and a sphere.

- Score the result.

2. *"Auditory" visualization*

- Mentally produce the sound of water dripping from a faucet or a running stream.

- Do the same with the sound of rhythmic ocean waves.
- Conjure up the sound of a familiar voice.
- Listen inwardly to a piece of instrumental music, and try to make out the different instruments.
- Give yourself a score for each instrument.

3. "Kinesthetic" visualization

- Tactile sensations: imagine that you pass your hand over the fur of a cat or dog, then the bark of a tree, followed by hot sand, and finally, snow.
- Kinesthetic sensation: try bending your right elbow in your imagination. Can you feel the physical sensation of the movement? Similarly, imagine you are holding a 10 kilo sack; then put it down, and be aware of someone shaking your hand.
- As before, evaluate your visualization on a scale of 1 to 10.

4. "Smelling and tasting" visualization

- Imagine the taste of a few foods or flavors (sweet, salty, bitter, sour, or acidic).
- Next imagine the smell of three or four scents (pleasant or unpleasant).
- What score did you give yourself for these sensory modalities?

5. Synthesis and applications

Your total score reveals your preferred sensory system. You might be comfortable with two or three ways of creatively imagining. Use your strong capacities for regular practice. Little by little, strengthen your weaker senses by visualizing with them every day for a week; then gradually decrease frequency. You may have noticed that some sense perceptions are easier in certain subcategories.

For example, the ability to see colors and faces references the emotional realm, while facility in viewing numbers and geometrical figures has more to do with one's mental register. In this way, you can discover if you are more familiar with the mental or emotional aspect of things.

Auditory pathways are more complex to analyze. If, when listening internally, your impressions are dominated by the ambiance of a sound (the tenor of nature, a babbling brook, or the sound of the sea, all of which are impressions linked to a tone of voice or atmospheric music), it means you register most of your impressions on the emotional wavelength. If, on the other hand, you vividly pick up the sound of running water, rolling waves, the spoken word or the rhythm and the parsing of music into notes and instruments, your nature is probably more mentally focused.

Here again, make best use of your natural abilities, while trying to develop other aspects. Repeat the exercise a few times, paying more attention to the dimensions that were less familiar to you the first time around.

The last point to consider is whether you find it easier to perceive and remain focused with your eyes open or closed? If the response is that you prefer your eyes open, you very certainly belong to the psychological type called "introvert."[1] In your case, impressions of your inner world are stronger than they are for the "extrovert," and dominate the outer world in your psychic economy. Nevertheless, with practice, introverted subjects can easily perform visualization with closed eyes. If you discover the answer is that you prefer your eyes closed because it is difficult for you to visualize with open eyes, you belong with the "extroverted" psychological type. This is because the impressions you take in from the surrounding world are so dominant that they interfere with your ability to concentrate and visualize internally.

Once you know your type, practice visualizing against type. This will expand your horizons.

[1] Jung, C. G., & Hull, R. F. C. (1991). *Psychological Types* (a revised ed.). London: Routlege.

When it comes to hearing, it is difficult to close off the ears. The use of noise-cancelling headphones is not a solution here. For the extrovert, learning to neutralize external noise can be very useful. Train yourself to perceive visually and auditorily next to a source of noise, such as a ticking alarm clock or conversation on the radio. It is possible to lose awareness of the external din, or at the very least have it lose all meaning, devolving into background noise. This amounts to hearing without listening.

In some instances, it can be helpful to imagine oneself in a bubble in order to help create a sense of insulation from the environment. This exercise is not recommended for those prone to daydreaming, or people who easily disconnect from their surroundings.

Not to be left out, I suggest this group try visualizing during concrete activities, such as knitting, crafts, manual tasks, or sports. Repeat the entire exercise in two or three months and compare any changes in your score. Are you satisfied with your progress?

Exercise 10: The safe place

This exercise is well known and generally much valued in psychotherapy. The objective is to learn to generate a positive internal state that you can easily recreate, no matter the circumstance. This ability is useful after a destabilizing, emotional episode, before approaching a delicate or sensitive situation, et cetera.

Sit comfortably with your eyes closed. (Eventually you will be able to do this exercise standing up in the middle of a crowd with your eyes open.) Imagine yourself in some real or imagined place that invokes in you, the epitome of *calm, serenity, and security.* This can be an enclosed space, such as a temple, church or house, or somewhere out in nature.

Take your time to imagine on your internal screen the general scene, filling in details, colors, ambient light, smells, and temperature. Use the sensory modalities that permit you to visualize most vividly. Experience yourself in this place on three levels.

- Physical: look for, feel, or imagine positive sensations.
- Emotional: look for, feel, or imagine positive feelings of calm, serenity, and security.
- Mental: think or imagine positive thoughts that associate with the location.

Indulge in this state for a while before returning to your regular day. Remember that, for the brain, the imagining of sensation, emotion, or thought is the same as the actual experience. Whatever is going on becomes the brain's reality in the moment. It is not a question of escaping some disturbing reality, but of being able to deal with it from a centered state that enables you to act in a constructive way.

Emotional incoherence

When the heart begins to speed up and pound away during an emotional event, it is a sign that we are more than a little off kilter, feeling disconnected from some part of ourselves. Our appraisal of a given situation that determines our emotional reaction to it can be at least:

- 50% influenced by the memory of similar situations we have lived through in the past;
- 50% influenced by our anticipation of what we risk by living in these disagreeable terms; and finally,
- a very small part of real evaluation of things.

Yes, that exceeds 100%, but this is precisely what our imagination is capable of when misapplied—adding more useless stuff than the situation warrants.

When we overreact, we are not fully in the moment, or operating from our true selves. This lack of self-awareness translates in practice to a perennial lack of confidence.

Experience has shown that when individuals are arbitrarily subjected to purely physiological stimulation of the systems that are activated during stress, they tend to look for an external cause to account for their symptoms. This helps explain how it is that we so often look outside ourselves to justify feeling miserable, making it difficult to evaluate situations accurately. Our responses and behavior are misaligned, almost as a matter of course, when we look to an external cause of the problem. Often we are not in the habit of self-empowerment.

Our emotions do not always (sometimes not at all) reflect the reality of situations. They then give rise to erroneous thoughts, which, in turn, reinforce the same emotional response. Here are some easily recognizable examples of inaccurate thinking.

- Dramatization
- Dichotomous thinking (where everything is black or white)
- Inappropriate generalization
- Excessive interpretation
- Hasty conclusion
- Impossible demands and perfectionism (I must absolutely; it has to be; if I do not do such and such, et cetera)
- Taking things personally
- Constant defensiveness and recurrent feelings of injustice

Exercise 11: Emotional control

How do you come back into balance and reconnect with yourself, after an emotion has thrown you askew? A good option is to proceed as follows.

- Recognize the emotion and name it ("I am angry," "I am afraid," for instance). It can be beneficial to verbalize your feeling to a third party, even if he or she is apparently the cause of your problem. Our emotions belong to us, and we should always feel responsible for our experiences. Are you not free to experience something else?
- Accept and welcome the emotion. This does not mean denying or repressing our feelings, and it does not

mean trying to get rid of the emotions—simply receive them. Reflect on the notion of welcoming them in general, and what a friendly or loving welcome means to you. You can greet your emotion, which, in the same vein, is to say "accept yourself." Rather than judging or condemning yourself thinking, "I did not want to be angry; what a terrible person I must be," acknowledge the way you reacted, while persevering in an effort to improve.

- Become centered in your body. Listen to what is going on. Notice how your breathing and heart rhythm react. Detect any sensations of tension or oppression that might have settled in some part of your body.
- Trust in the process without looking to control it, an attitude that generally produces the opposite effect. Let it be.
- Assess the nature of the situation. Take a step back and check to see if your apprehension is well founded, and determine what is reasonably possible to do or not do.
- The above steps afford us, in cases that are not too thorny, the liberty to alter our state of being and, in the final analysis, be more equitable to ourselves and others. Try out the experience.

For example, the next time you feel agitation building up inside, go over these six steps.

1. Before allowing yourself to explode with anger, for instance, pause for a second to give yourself the option of living differently. Say words to the effect of, "Hey, I'm angry; well it's not the first time."

2. Accept that anger is part of what it means to be human. The challenge is to become the subject of this anger by directing and transforming the feeling to our benefit. Do not repress the feeling or behave as if the anger does not exist. It is of no help to lie to yourself

or others. This only works against you in one way or another, which may turn up later as psychosomatic symptoms. Neither should you let off steam or become preoccupied with whomever you feel is responsible for keeping you trapped in anger. This is of no advantage to yourself or to them. Accept yourself, just as you are, in the moment.

3. Perceive how tensions arise in the muscles of your back, neck, and jaw; observe that your breathing becomes more rapid and superficial.

4. Have faith in your capacity to change, to evolve, and simply "to be."

5. Analyze what exactly happened to make you so angry (rather than to focus on who made you angry). Replay the film from the beginning. Try to see where things went off the rails without passing judgment of the other person's rationale. Or at the very least, consider the actions and the words involved, not just the one who committed or uttered them.

Exercise 12: The Buddha smile

This exercise is designed to accomplish the same result as the above, but in a more direct and immediate way. The mental image of a smile can produce a positive state of detachment in the midst of a stressful situation.

- Allow yourself to become aware of whatever emotional agitation has arisen. Center your attention on the sounds of the body's typical stress response: clenching, palpitations, rapid and shallow breathing, and so on.

- Smile inwardly "to yourself," conjuring up all its positive connotations: calmness, quietude, and serenity, physically as much as emotionally and mentally. The goal is to *choose* to instill a positive internal state. You can find inspiration for such detachment and composure by gazing at Buddha's smile, illustrated in Figure 15. Equanimity is by no means synonymous with indifference. Evenness of mind simply implies the calm and benevolent understanding of one who has risen above the grievances and more childish aspect of the human personality, called our *ego*.

- Practice a few rounds of *coherent breathing* into the heart center, clearing away any inharmonious thoughts, feelings, or sensations with each exhalation.
- Give free rein to this inner state and resolve to maintain it as you return to the external situation at hand. With practice, it will be possible to come back to center in a matter of minutes.

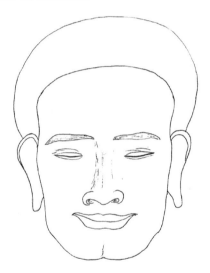

Figure 15. The Buddha smile.

Before applying this exercise for real, run through it several times with reference to some recent upheaval. Place yourself back in the context of an irritating situation until you feel the same feelings arise. It is not in the least way harmful to recreate negative emotions artificially. They are, after all, latent within us, registered in the brain. Revisiting them can reduce their future potency. If you cannot easily revive the feeling, act as though you have, and the effect will be the same. The gap between recapturing the sensation and imagining you have recaptured it is less than you imagine.

Desires

Albeit that the brain operates as a function of our sociocultural conditioning, this does not excuse us from being responsible for our faltering nature. Each of us collaborates in self-fulfillment through our desires. We want a beautiful house, new clothes, the latest electronics, a wife or husband, car, and dog. Even laudable public spirited accomplishments can be—admittedly commendable—sources of love, recognition, ease, and comfort. Even the inclination to be magnanimous can have this same underlying quality. I do not mean to imply that good and charitable individuals look to be rewarded. But an overly pronounced yearning to be good and charitable can lead one to suspect this centripetal tendency matches some need. In summary, the key word and the impetus of many behaviors is *having*.

Lest the reader take me for an embittered moralist prone to advocating abstinence and privation, none of these things are bad in and of themselves. The source of our difficulties lies in our lack of freedom in relationship to such things, our inability to be autonomous with regard to situations, relationships, and objects we possess, or desire to possess. *We let our happiness depend on things rather than on ourselves.*

It is said that money cannot buy happiness, and that the world is full of rich and unhappy people. "Having" does not create happiness either; it provides only satisfaction.

Satisfaction is essentially ephemeral, a condition that must be constantly replenished. The demands of gratification tend to steadily increase in order that the same level of pleasure and contentment be attained. The paradoxical challenge is to know how to enjoy passing fulfillments without being dependent on them, and to maintain stable internal integrity when external provisions are lacking.

Only *being* is permanent. Its nature is to radiate, like the sun. To be in touch with our true nature is to sit beside an inexhaustible source, where *love* and *joy* grow in us beyond the reach of the tribulations that inevitably mark our existence.

Exercise 13: Unfolding desires

The goal of the following exercise is to make us aware of our connection to *having* in order to better tap into our demand for *being*. You will have to discover the current underlying desire, that is to say, what motivates it. Then discover the first impulse that lies even deeper. Keep this in mind during the exercise.

First phase of the exercise

Sitting comfortably, focus on something you want at present, but one that is problematic in some way or another. If no such desire comes to mind, any past fancy or desire will work, as long as you have already had the satisfaction of fulfilling it.

Bring this strong wish to the fore as clearly as possible. Imagine all the nuances; every thought, word, and deed required in the quest, whatever it may be. Try to perceive, in as much detail as possible, *the state of psychic tension* leading up to the desire coming true.

Bring to mind all the "feelings" associated with achieving what you want. To take a trivial example, set your heart on a delicious lemon meringue tart. Visualize it in all its delectable detail, reliving the feeling brought on by peering through the pastry shop window, seeing yourself entering the shop, and buying the tart. Salivate at the very sight of the dessert before you even bite into it. Finally, revel in the consistency and the different flavors you taste in your mouth.

Indulge your senses to the fullest. However, keep in mind that the purpose here is not creative fantasies or psychic gratification, only a preliminary introduction to reimagining true life incidents.

Repeat the experience, keeping a parallel sense of the attendant pressures or tension associated with the desire before it was met, and the feelings related to the experience of satisfaction. Feel free to use the memories of similar experiences you have known.

Are there any slight differences between the two phases? Does the satisfaction of the desire match up to the expectations of the initial urge? Is it an exact equivalent? Does it carry a feeling of plenitude?

In analyzing the perceived anticipatory pressures, you will doubtless discover that a level of quiet dissatisfaction remains. This residual feeling has become, for some, a standard part of daily life. This quiet dissatisfaction drives us in steady search of new sources of indulgence.

Focus for a minute on this subtle feeling of discontent. Identify and intensify the nature of it. You may discover something less well defined than the wish to consume a defined object. A more vital sense of *need,* something on the order of a *vacuum* that seeks to be filled—an existential *lack.* This vague sense of the unattainable informs our life with such force that no satisfaction can ever really silence it. We are, by nature, wanting beings, or so it would appear. How many lives have been broken, ruined on the shoals of some perceived shortfall? However, this same sense of "not enough" is a formidable source of human creativity and purpose. Art, literature, science, religion, and architecture are all indebted to an underlying absence that feeds human genius. Once the relentless quest for material need is met, a perception that there is something more, becomes the driving force of human ingenuity and higher aspirations.

Here we discover an inner spark that seeks expression. We ourselves give shape and direction to this energy by offering it receptacles that transform it into desires, then satisfaction. The choice of containers, their form and management, is generally what leads us to be happy or unhappy.

Become familiar with this exercise by applying it to various desires. When you feel you have managed to identify the undercurrent of desire, proceed to the second phase.

Second phase of the exercise

The next step is to directly perceive the sense of vital yearning, the lack of which presides over desire. Become as aware as possible of desire and its undercurrent during the course of your life. It is as if you descend more deeply within and deal with this need.

Delve in a little farther still in search of what motivates this demand, something a little upstream. This phase is more difficult than the first, and please do not become discouraged if the awaited perception does not appear. It requires more elaborate internal work. Any effort you put in will produce effects, even if they remain unconscious. Keep a relaxed mental attitude, and do not try to force perception.

With time, you may be able to anticipate a first impulse, the motivator that underlies even basic need. This inclination relates to the transition from *having* to *being,* from the personal to the impersonal. We contact the very heart of the human being. The vital and fundamental impulse of being is a centrifugal, not a centripetal energy; it is a radiating, not a taking, energy. The question changes from "How to have?" to "What to be?" The quality of being is to exist and shine, like the sun. This is also the metaphor of *love.*

Cultivate this state of being—the exercise offers a way to move in this direction—and you will find your life "enlarged."

Interlude

Cultivate as much good humor and laughter as you can on a daily basis. Laughter is a wonderful medicine. It causes us to secrete youth hormones, relaxes diaphragmatic muscle tension, and much more.

We owe it to our loved ones to communicate the joy and cheerfulness that comes through in day to day good humor and lightheartedness. Looking sullen, morose, or irritable is a form of violence towards others, something that will reverberate back to us in one form or another.

Raising good natured children guarantees their healthy development, and immunizes them from the effects of stress. To be positively childish is ultimately far less infantile than taking oneself too seriously or giving in to every emotion.

3 ⌒

Mental equilibrium

Preamble

As a species, our collective mental state has undergone tremendous development over the past two centuries. Rising global literacy rates, together with advances in education, have brought a colossal increase in access to information. The mind, already the most recent structure in our evolution, is still in the early stages of development, and far from having reached its full potential. Moreover, it is believed that we use only a small percentage of our brain capacity.

We will see in pages to come that our thoughts, some dearly held ideas, and opinions that we stubbornly cling to are not as freely held and self-determined as all that. Many people are victims of mental agitation, fixed ideas, or runaway ruminations of which they frequently complain. This absence of liberty concerning our thoughts is responsible for confusion, absence of mental clarity, poor decisions, loss of motivation, and insomnia. Apparently, women are statistically more "gifted" at lying awake, pondering problems, but we don't put much faith in statistics.

A dynamic mind is never agitated or overly worked up, despite it being more active and many times more effective. A sprightly mind allows us to plan, learn, work, create, comprehend clearly, and embark on a project, all in less time and using less energy than its flustered, overwrought counterpart.

A human being cannot find balance without being level-headed. If emotional balance occurs through "elimination" and the alleviation of negative emotional charges, then the management of our "mental body" is partly due to it having been educated and it being given a purpose. An enlightened, structured mind, built up little by little, counterbalances the tyranny of our emotions. It increases our capacity for insight and perspective, and contributes to our freedom. It is this aspect that we will now address.

Our personality, the "self" psychologists speak of, is made up of our physical body, our emotional field, and the realm of our thoughts or thought field. The personality, as such, possesses both innate and acquired characteristics. Several factors contribute to shaping our character include:

- hereditary tendencies, connected to the type and distinctive features of our physical body;
- the influence of our childhood family circle, in terms of the emotional and mental temperament of our parents, their expectations of us, the conscious and unconscious issues they passed on—in short, intersubjective elements that occur between two separate conscious minds, thoroughly described by psychoanalysts;
- sociocultural and national influences of the country we grew up inform the basis of our social, racial, and nationalistic prejudices, contributing to our worldview in ways we hardly realize; and
- important personal events: various separations, emotional shocks, bereavements, illnesses, accidents, and the like.

All these influences are well in the past. Can we alter even one iota of what happened long ago? Evidently not.

How many patients have I met over the years who have many hours of psychotherapy behind them, and yet seem incapable of leading a balanced and fulfilling life? What is the reason for this major failing, common to most forms of psychotherapy? Analyzing the past as it relates to current situations, seems justifiable in the first part of adult life, when it can help people find their way. Some individuals do not have an easy time fitting in socially or professionally, and others find even normal emotional relationships difficult. Such pathological challenges can happily be identified, acknowledged, and understood through psychotherapy.

Nevertheless, in many cases the pitfall of psychotherapy is that it feeds past torments and certain personality dysfunctions that are marked by the short comings and excesses of life experience. The mental habit of regularly looking into erstwhile events can lead to several consequences, among them:

- tuning our attention to our suffering and failings (the glass-is-half-empty, scenario);
- reinforcing the idea that our past justifies current problems ("Some things cannot change; I am what I am.");
- justifying weaknesses in character;
- encouraging complacency and self-pity; and
- leading to perpetual demands that things be put right, in the form of asking for amends from others and society, if not the entire world.

The latter eventuality is perhaps the worst of all, in that it squelches any possibilities of becoming a self-sufficient person, someone able to create his own happiness. Such a person will not easily cease from demanding his due from all quarters, distorting his relationship to life and other people. We can see the increasingly large part this irresponsible attitude plays in modern society. Reparations are commonly claimed for everything and anything, an attitude supported by lawyers who see the possibility of healthy remuneration. People believe they can escape their anxieties and health problems, so often difficulties they themselves helped create, through compensation awarded by the courts.

Psychotherapists must be vigilant in such scenarios and persevere in supporting the psychic autonomy of their patients.

Treatment that continues for years has little chance of fitting this objective.

It is necessary to recognize psychotherapeutic streams that work towards restoring human dignity, through either a higher form of personality integration or the fostering of an individual's innate healing abilities. Humanistic psychology and self-actualization therapies are two examples. On the other hand, mankind wanting to repair his ego is like a person trying to levitate; it is impossible, and sometimes grotesque to even imagine.

The serenity prayer by Reinhold Niebuhr puts it this way: "My God, give us the grace to accept with serenity the things that cannot be changed, courage to change the things that should be changed, and the wisdom to distinguish the one from the other."

Possibilities for revision and for building a happy and fulfilling life do most certainly exist. It is not a matter of wanting to alter what is no longer amenable, nor of struggling in vain against our defects and weaknesses, but rather of cultivating what is good, just, and constructive.

Oriental sages have never proclaimed anything different; their methods always accentuate the positive. Instead of advising disciples to, "Rid yourself of what is impure," they advise, "Do your best to acquire greater purity, and the impurities will dissolve by themselves. Do not fight to cast away darkness, but put on the light, and the gloom will disappear."

Darkness represents the part of us that is underdeveloped and unable to grow harmoniously, because we are by nature imperfect, and human evolution is not yet complete. Our imperfection is reinforced by all the traumatic ups and downs or deficiencies of our existence. To investigate this darkness from every angle, determining whether it is linked to mother, father, or our long deceased great-great grandmother (whose psycho-genealogical imprint we still bear) often sheds no light. At best we can become aware that if darkness intensifies in some situations, it is simply wiser to steer clear of them.

Another approach is to do just the opposite, and allow the brighter part of ourselves to come forth. This more luminous potential is carried deep within. It is the essence and the promise of the true human being, something we shall refer to here as the *self*. Regardless of our philosophical or religious views, whether we believe in a soul, some divine principle, or are atheistic, history bears ample traces of human beings who have actualized this *self* to a very high degree as a testament to the best and greatest man can be. The only condition is that we believe in mankind's potential and, therefore, in the most luminous part of ourselves, our deeper *self* or spiritual nature.

Trust that you hold the promise of a just, happy, serene, and fulfilling existence. Have faith that your inner light can dissolve darkness, no matter your personal narrative. Some call this *resilience,* the ability to spring back from difficult conditions.

Exercise 14: Relaxation

The principles of this exercise are widely used in various relaxation methods. The way we teach it here, beyond offering profound physical relaxation, is meant to enhance mindfulness. A calm and clear mind is centered and able to focus in whatever direction the subject guides it. An attentive mind is also a relaxed mind. This is one of the most delightful routines presented in this book. We recommend you repeat it daily, or at least three times a week, for as long as you like.

This practice is done lying comfortably on your back, at least the first time around. Later you can do it sitting up and, if necessary, a little faster. Fifteen minutes is a good average time period to start with.

Principle

Focus your attention on your right foot. This can be done in different ways, depending on your favorite sensory style. You can feel your foot, "look inside," or a combination of the two. The main thing is to keep your attention on this part of the body. If you don't find this easy, content yourself with imagining that you feel or see it, and the result will be more or less the same. The idea is to move your awareness gradually up the leg, as far as the pelvis, and then proceed as follows.

- Completely relax the part of the lower limb on which you are focused. Then move up the leg to the next zone, leaving the relaxed part completely inert, without any activity. You can also imagine that the relaxed part "goes out" and becomes dark, with no activity or tension.
- Move up the leg little by little, bringing the light of the relaxed part into the next zone. This light then goes off as you move your focus up your leg, and so on up to the pelvis. You gradually "turn off" your entire lower limb, bringing light (or activity) back to the pelvis.

The exercise in stages
- Relax the entire right lower limb: foot, ankle, leg, calf, knee, thigh, and hip.
- Relax the entire left lower limb, as above.
- Relax the entire right upper limb: fingers, hand, wrist, forearm, elbow, arm, and shoulder.
- Relax the entire left upper limb, as above.
- Relax the trunk. Begin at the pelvis, your "foundation," and move up gradually: abdomen, lumbar spine, diaphragm, ribcage, thoracic spine, throat, neck, and cervical column. The diaphragm is the only muscle that you cannot render inert. Simply become aware of its movement during breathing. Allow the entire trunk to become inert and tension free, "switched off."
- Relax your face, jaw, and brow.
- Internalization. This is the final and all-important part of the exercise.
- Enter the very center your head with all the light you brought to the rest of your body. Become aware of a

central luminous point, and do your best to be entirely focused on this place.

- Internalize your view, imagining that you can see inside of yourself with your eyes closed. From the central point, imagine that you see into another dimension, a space different from what presently surround you physically. Use your creative vision.
- Next, internalize your sense of hearing, sense of smell, and finally of taste, proceeding in the same manner.
- Remain in this state a few minutes to benefit from the new and special consciousness. See, hear, feel, and taste the Presence within you.

The only caution is to please not fall into a state of such passivity that your thoughts wander aimlessly. Remain attentive, master of your reverie.

The mental culture

The levels of consciousness

Our consciousness encompasses all ideas, emotions, impressions, and sensations that we are aware of at any given moment. It is what we perceive as our sense of selfhood.

Below the conscious threshold lies the subconscious. In this vast reservoir, dwell countless realms of impressions, associations, and conceptions, informed by **everything** that has been recorded since our birth, consciously or unconsciously. Subconscious material can easily spill into the conscious mind. It is enough to think of something for that something to come to consciousness, occasionally bringing with it impressions that are in some way related.

Sometimes these elements are brought to consciousness without us having any idea what brought them into our awareness—a slip of the tongue, for example.

Everything that is available for recall and capable of becoming conscious Freud termed *the preconscious*. Each person is endowed with a fairly extensive and functional preconscious. Psychoanalysts speak of the *depth* and the *permeability of the preconscious,* the innumerable thoughts or memories that relate in part to an individual's imagination.

Vaster still than Freud's notion of the subconscious is the concept of the unconscious, to which thousands of books have been devoted and still not plumbed its full extent, which might as well be as infinite as the universe. Nevertheless, its effects on the human psyche make it something we can study and understand, if only to a degree.

The main thing about which everyone seems to agree is the crucial role the unconscious mind plays in behavior, judgment, and emotion. It influences our lives, motivation, choices, and personality features informing the ideas and opinions we hold.

In the modern era in which we make strong claims to individual freedom in all facets of our existence, we have not yet, it would seem, calculated that our so-called liberty is in fact stolen away, and the tyrant is within us.

Honest reflection would take into account the obvious. Much of what we like or detest, our hopes, desires, personal tastes, opinions and fears, inhibitions, and so much more have not been entirely chosen by ourselves. What is more we cannot quite say why and how all these things are as they are. Among the unconscious processes that affect us, some are of little consequence to our lives, while others cast limits or have a destructive and corrupting influence, sometimes to detrimental outcome. Winning our true freedom, meaning self-determination and psychic autonomy, requires first that we be willing to accept the extent of unconscious phenomena within us. Once we understand how these elements function in our psyche, we can engage with them, and by gradually neutralizing them, gain better command over our lives.

Complexes

A complex is a group of psychic elements united around a highly charged affective mental or psycho-emotional core. All emotions, memories, and impressions received since childhood are stored in our subconscious. Deeply ingrained are our family environment, education, and the psycho-emotional climate that nourished us, the socio-cultural milieu in which we have grown up and continue to evolve opinions, beliefs, and sense of belonging. These all add up to an extraordinary combination of rich and pertinent imprints, blended with a jumble of beliefs, conventional wisdom, superstition, dogma, fictions, and illusions.

Our media-saturated era grows increasingly sophisticated, further complicating the economy of our intrapsychic complexes. We allow millions of images to penetrate us every day, and hundreds of bits of information stick to our complexes. Some people are inclined to develop certain complexes by their very disposition. For example, a person with worry and anxious tendencies will be especially receptive to images and information related to disasters, crimes, and other incivilities, leading to distorted thoughts about how dangerous the world is— a fear complex.

Each of us carries in his subconscious numerous complexes collected around themes of a mental or emotional nature, or very often a blend of the two. We lead our lives under the auspice of the unconscious mind that is possessed of an unsuspected strength. Depending on the complex, this force can be positive or negative, a help or a hindrance in life.

The main thing to grasp is that a complex is a distorted way of thinking that operates automatically, mechanically, and instinctively. It needs only to be fed regularly to grow and strengthen. Here we find a functional vicious circle is at play. *All complexes focus mental and emotional awareness on whatever resonates with the complex, which in turn becomes steadily enlivened by the attention.*

Worries and ruminations are generally nothing more than the activation of a complex at work. They represent continuous thoughts that self-replicate, without any opportunity for relevant change that might lead to a constructive result. A seemingly interminable list of negative complexes includes: guilt, shame, prejudice, phobias, fixed ideas, anxiety, and inferiority or superiority complexes.

Complexes generally run counter to a fulfilling life, and their activation can incline us to believe that we are powerless to change: "I can't help the way I am." Our will seems too weak. This is the moment our loss of freedom begins.

Self-determination can seem a daunting task, and while it might involve a very gradual conquest, it is not unattainable. Gaining control over our life requires that we overcome the biases, fictions, and illusions of our conditioning, and find nourishment from other sources. This requires some daring— the bravery to cultivate other values and aspirations, to be open to a new inner listening, and to the sounds of *life* and *being* that only await our call to infuse our existence.

Western society, which is immersed, has its own genius, qualities, and knowledge, from which the entire world has benefited. Nevertheless, it has its own demons, not the least of which is an arrogance and sense of superiority in relation to other cultures. We denounce, sometimes with good reason, the indoctrination of people, particularly children in countries where sectarianism and fundamentalism flourish. But are we really any less conditioned in our countries? The media sets the pace of the mass culture. Our freedom of thought is further limited to whatever part of the political spectrum we belong, the religion we follow, the view on war and peace we hold, and any number of things with which we choose to identify—be it an atheist or believer, radical or conservative, agitator or peacenik. Liberty is admittedly precious, but must be weighed in the balance against the notion that we have not been entirely free in the unfolding of our personal conditioning that leads to our present choices.

Who can say that he would not have blown himself up in the middle of a crowd if fate had not placed him in a hapless group of martyrs (blessed by his tutors) who believe in the promise of paradise for his heroic act of murder? We also wholeheartedly defend and rise to the defense of what we see as great causes whose outcome is perceived as pivotal to national prestige and honor.

Modern Western culture has an interesting but singular secret. It leads us toward a maniac individualism by acting through the lever of collectivism. To our misfortune, these "isms" are often distorted, when in fact both possess the ingredients for true happiness:

Individualism, in the sense of egoism, is an "every man for himself" attitude. It insists, "I have the right," or "the community (society, state, another person) owes me." This, unfortunately, usurps a truer individuality that is founded on the ability to choose and think for oneself—to be original. It is the freedom to write or behave as one wishes, even in a politically incorrect manner. Collectivism is the sense of a collective bias concerning what is commendable, admirable, and good to have (and not to have, to be more accurate) in order to be "happy." All this is instead of a feeling of belonging and fraternity, love and altruism—the true spirit of one for all, and all for one.

Have you ever noticed that the happiest people are those who do not search like maniacs for what is called *happiness*? Nowadays happiness tends to mean satisfying the senses, and giving free reign to our emotions, bringing us back to our discussion of *having*.

Happy are the people who place their priority on *being*. Such beings rarely sit in centripetal energy, a vibration that perpetually draws things their way. On the contrary, they participate in centrifugal movement, the free flow and distribution of what they do and are. Perhaps they do not know modern happiness, but nevertheless rejoice. Unlike happiness, joy is not ephemeral.

Try to see the practical opportunities of cultivating your mind in a healthy and constructive way, that you might escape the attraction of negative complexes that tend to govern us. This is doubtless the most difficult part of the work proposed in this book. All the preceding exercises are designed to help you approach this section by improving your powers of concentration, and the capacity to direct your attention at will.

Exercise 15: Developing attention

This exercise involves paying attention to whatever is happening from moment to moment. It can be done any time, any place, whenever you have a few quiet moments to spare. Begin by devoting a short time in the evening before bed, as it is an excellent way to avoid insomnia brought on by ruminations. The principle is simple: be present to everything that comes across your field of consciousness, without any attempt to control, direct, or censor material.

It is important that you remain mindful, but without the slightest tension of effort. Watch your thoughts unfold as if you were glancing absent-mindedly at a television. Assume the *attitude of an observer.*

Learn to make out the origin of your thoughts. Do they arise because of some external element, perhaps a recent situation, some topic related to incidents in your life, or are they prompted by current events from the news media? Could they derive from a deeper and more intimate part of you, perhaps from your subconscious?

Next, ask yourself if anything new comes forward, and if these thoughts are transformed or modified in some way or other as they transit through your field of consciousness. If so, in what sense? What was the job of your unconscious? Was it a screen on which thoughts appear, or a crucible in which what is put inside is stirred together, associated, or transformed in some way?

You will soon perceive that this simple act of paying attention to your thoughts automatically filters negative or no longer useful thoughts, emotions, and impressions. This feature of the mind brings peacefulness, calm, and clarity. Discontinue the exercise as soon as fatigue or tension set in, and practice relaxation exercise 14, if you feel so inclined.

Pathways to freedom

Since time immemorial, human beings have sought to alleviate suffering. Over centuries, the Judeo-Christian civilization has attempted to elevate itself by highlighting moral values in combination with the eradication of vices and sins. While the spiritual essence of these religions is beyond criticism, history shows that their exponents have not always been shining examples of lives lived in the virtuous way their religion espouses.

The arrival of psychoanalysis at the dawn of the twentieth century brought a revolution to the understanding and care of the human soul. There were many, and legion more today, who believed they had finally found the whys and wherefores of the vulnerability and hidden nature of the psyche. In as much as the study of psychoanalytic theory is fascinating, equally intriguing are its disappointing therapeutic results, such as years of therapy devoted to understanding the origin of neurosis. Too often, the greatest beneficiary of the many hours spent spinning circles around the bleaker points of any psychic disorder is the psychological affliction itself.

Psychoanalysis went on to produced numerous branches that combined theories from many sources, to the extent that today the list of different schools is rather spectacular. The common denominator is the near sacred focus these schools place on the emotional aspect, echoing current societal values. On one hand is the tradition that stifled emotional memories need to be expressed, while on the other, a belief that a steady supply of pleasurable emotion is a requirement for ongoing happiness, or an emotional sentimentality in which tears are seen as the height of compassion.

So common is the prevailing therapeutic view that those who speak out against it can be labeled as cold, cerebral, or insensitive. Yet, oftentimes the more attention that is focused on the emotional, the more negative emotions are amplified in the imagination. This muddies our thoughts and interferes with our ability to make choices with creativity of purpose, which otherwise would provide some glimmer of peace, serenity, and lasting contentment.

We routinely operate in ways that drive and reinforce complexes that are hostile to our well-being. Excessive emotional focus, with the deliberate intention of resolving or repenting for things past, can leave us complacent, sad, or ashamed of our faults and perceived personal weaknesses. The mere act of steadily paying attention to complexes energizes and complexifies them.

The secret to weakening our complexes is so simple that it tends to meet with distain among intellectuals who theorize about the psyche. The key is to enfeeble the complex through undernourishment. If a complex is not replenished, it will eventually lose its power of attraction and influence over our consciousness. Through patience and determination, it is enough to stop paying attention to strong emotionally-colored thoughts.

Not all complexes have the same power over us, and some are more difficult to deactivate than others. At first, you may encounter resistance, sometimes even a transient worsening of disharmony. With perseverance and sincerity, you are certain to succeed. Fake it until you make it.

Reflect honestly on your genuineness. We can often be more attached to certain of our faults than others, generally those that appear to bring us more pleasure than annoyance. But benefits of this type are illusory, and tend to catch up with us sooner or later.

Similarly, it is necessary to fortify our mental field. Avoid confusing the mental field with "things cerebral," or cool, calculated intellectualism. The mind is the field in which our thoughts unfold clearly, efficiently, and in an intelligent way. The mental field encompasses life intelligence, not just intelligence quotient (I.Q.). The mind holds the power to refashion our lives though inner transformation.

A verse from the Upanishad puts it this way, "However a man thinketh, he is." This works both ways. If you believe yourself to be incompetent, angry, virtuous, or capable, you can remain so, or become that way, if you are not already.

We can break with the eternal refrain "change is impossible" and instead re-construct our personality to suit ourselves better. Our most powerful tool for this is the same that we involuntarily use to limit ourselves—the imagination. Through creative vision, we can form new complexes, or what might be called positive counter-complexes, that is, patterns of thought that help move us in our desired direction. Creative imagination requires only the help of mindfulness and a well-directed will.

Fairly soon, old complexes will be blocked by counter complexes that act automatically and mechanically. They attract what is in harmonic resonance with our nature, dissolving negative thoughts and emotions with which we are no longer in alignment. Outdated complexes will thus be disabled, without the need to dwell on their origin or symbolic significance. Let us now look at how this might happen.

Exercise 16: Complex de-activation and activation

Take a moment to study your personality, your character, and make a list of your most common faults and weaknesses. Do not be too hard on yourself and avoid listing forty defects. Minor short-comings do not even merit consideration, as they are only aspects that add flourish to our individuality, and not something we take too seriously. Hold just two or three imperfections in your mind, for it will not be possible to focus on several at once. Then evacuate them out of your mind—definitely!

Keep your focus, and meditate on the opposite quality or some virtue that you wish to enhance in your character. Form a clear picture of all the effects and consequences that this new addition will bring to your life. Test out how this virtue feels in yourself, in both body and spirit.

Sense the tone of the emotional state that arises. Create a new resonance in your mind and body, and slowly your entire being will change.

Pay close attention to this quality for several minutes each morning, never missing a day. Mental configuration is something fragile at the beginning, and must be sustained regularly. Negative complexes carve their path overtime. Patterns of distorted emotion, thought, and perception require patience to erase and replace. Such a process must continue for some time before risk of relapse passes. Just how long this takes depends on how strong and ingrained the complex might be, your aptitude for mindfulness, and the depth of your desire and willingness to be recreated.

In any event, there are bound to be some setbacks early on in the endeavor. Do not let this concern you, and avoid self-judgment. Simply tell yourself something along the lines of: "I wanted to do better; it has not been easy, but I hope to make headway next time." Be patient. The venture has begun. Continue to imagine yourself as you wish to be, and soon it will be so.

The mind can only turn in one direction at a time. If you set your intention on replacing all negative thoughts with their opposites, the former will occupy less of your mind to the benefit of more positive elements. You will cease from struggling against what no longer sits right with you.

With more tenacious negative thoughts and emotions, the trick is to find a short phrase that expresses the opposite thought or emotion—something to be repeated each time the negative aspect presents itself. This may remind you of the Coué method of autosuggestion, by which repeating words or images is enough to cause the subconscious to absorb them and thereby change our inner world. These principles are not as simplistic as general opinion would have it. Here we go beyond reframing affirmations.

The methodical application of the principles that you have been taught in this book is an inventive approach to our mental field. This can bring forth the volitional "I," capable of directing its will and become self-determined. The criticism that it might be no more than simply autosuggestion does not hold water because, after all, we live in a constant state of autosuggestion from what we have absorbed over a lifetime. Even in this case, why not switch from negative autosuggestion to one that enhances well-being, liberty, and creativity of purpose?

Exercise 17: Positive attitude

The accumulation of negative thoughts is the worst poison a human being is capable of inflicting on himself. Criticism of ourselves or others amount to the same thing, and only ends up immersing us in a pointless and unproductive atmosphere, nurtured by precisely what it is we criticize.

It is wise to be aware that our discontent and irritation about everything and nothing, and our relentless judgment contribute to the negative mental and emotional mood of the collective unconscious. We ought to feel the responsibility to offer the world, or at least our immediate circle, the best of ourselves. Unconsciously, what we reproach in others or where we find fault in society at large is often a part of ourselves that we do not recognize, and seeing it mirrored in others is intolerable. Constant fault finding is a sign of pride, and generates nothing but conflict.

Apart from life-threatening situations, most human quarrels can be resolved, if you accept that changing others is not necessarily possible, and take responsibility for yourself. There is always a part in you that arouses or maintains discord. How you react is up to you. If someone annoys you, it is you that empowers their actions or words to exasperate you. You are the sole keeper of your inner balance, and demanding the world conform to your expectations will leave you perennially dissatisfied.

By creating harmony within, peace and tranquility will grow around you, as you naturally attract what resonates with your inner state.

What is the best way to ward off negativity? Systematically train yourself to pay attention to what is good, just, and beautiful in those you encounter in your day, neglecting on *principle* their trespasses and flaws. Notice only their merits.

For those of you prone to self-devaluation, treat yourself the same way. Become an expert in voluntarily forgetting the dark side of human nature, so that it may be devitalized. This is true tolerance.

Become adept at finding attributes that, with a little effort, it is possible to discern in everyone. Reinforce what is positive in those around you. Living this way, your own life becomes a model, modest as it is.

Until this disposition becomes completely natural, take a few minutes each evening to review your personal interactions earlier that day. In your imagination, restore positive relations and feel the appreciation you might have had for someone, if a negative outlook had not contributed to an unfriendly atmosphere.

Mental function

Embarking on the following exercises may bring an initial sense of increased mental agitation. This is because we are not accustomed to placing this form of mental pressure on our mind, or feeling the reaction to this exertion.

In physics and psychology, laws governing energy and forces have a tendency to bring everything towards a zero degree of tension. This state of zero tension is the state of greatest stability, but it is also a static state, the enemy of movement in any complex form of organization. It represents nothingness and death, while paradoxically, supreme comfort.

How our universe could have been created from nothingness and then expand into complex forms like galaxies, stars, planets, and then biological life is a fascinating physical and metaphysical question that physicians, philosophers, and religious systems have long considered. Man, being the fruit of this universe, does not escape its laws and the energies that ceaselessly mobilize and bring new things into existence, at least for the time being. The law of cycles, of alternating activity and rest, of existence in this form, and then the death of the same human form creates an energetic struggle between being and non-being, between what we know of as *life* and *death*.

Our mind is not free of forces that can, at different times, prompt it into work, cause inaction, or produce chaotic functioning. We sometimes feel this as laziness.

The mental "pressure" induced by focusing exercises interrupts the established order of things. Nevertheless, in a matter of weeks, short lived agitation falls into a new order, and harmony is restored.

There is another explanation for the initial feeling of mental agitation. The mind that is unaccustomed to focus is already quite stirred up. Meditation brings awareness to this turmoil, which has, until now, carried on just beneath the veil of consciousness. The goal of building healthy mental clarity is to be able to increase concentration when required, and reduce useless activity when no mental effort is needed.

A clear mind is able to reflect on the essentials of a problem, and then effectively organize and put into effect a possible solution. Such a mind relaxes when all that needs to be done has been accomplished. It is able to let go of ruminations that tend to turn over old ground, when not channeled towards an immediate task. An undomesticated mind is marked by the repetition compulsion.

Exercise 18: Concentration

This exercise is best practiced in the evening, before bed.

Part one

Choose as a focus some current preoccupation or project that requires all your faculties to resolve or complete. Center your awareness and attention in the heart region, as you learned to do in the preliminary exercises.

Breathe fully, deeply, and rhythmically. Without tension, focus your mind on the chosen topic. Depending on the situation, conjure up all aspects of the matter, searching for any novel detail. In this state of meditation, it is not unusual for a fresh clarity to appear. It may be the next morning that a new idea spontaneously turns up, your mind having worked on the problem unconsciously through the night. Remain physically and mentally disengaged. Do not force yourself to try to understand more, but instead allow the higher mental resources to work.

Each time that your mind wanders astray, gently bring it back to center. Proceed to conjure up solutions, and plan what must be done in the coming days.

Part two: "Stop thinking!"

As soon as you are satisfied with your meditation and feel that nothing new is likely to shown up for the moment, or your thoughts are tending to repeat themselves, try relinquishing all thoughts. This is naturally a little more difficult to do, as it runs contrary to the nature of our mind. Zero mental tension does not mean going blank. It is a chaos of thoughts that follow each other without order and reproduce themselves endlessly.

Proceed patiently, clearing away each thought as it presents itself. Imagine the emptiness, with a symbol of your choice. A few seconds without thought has astonishing restorative effects. In most cases, this state does not last very long. It is a fleeting parenthesis, a way station to other things, but the experience is unforgettable.

The absence of thoughts is not the absence of awareness. It is an altered state, in which we are no more centered in our mind than we are in our emotions. It is a physical and psychic realm of consciousness, whose center is non-localized. It resembles the stillness of the mystic ecstatics, or the limitless serenity of nirvana, a place at the entryway to transcending human consciousness.

Here, only your personal encounter has any meaning. I can only invite you to enter into the experience; the rest is up to you.

Conclusion

We have arrived at the end of the book. On first reading, you might feel daunted by the number of exercises, or think the whole thing calls for altogether too much discipline and effort. These impressions are natural, and due largely to a misreading of the time factor, and perhaps misdirection of the imagination. Rome was not built in a day, and man cannot be remade in a short time. This book is not a recipe for a miracle, and it can promise nothing more than what you can give yourself. Learn to repurpose the imagination in a creative direction, instead of leaving it in a static state that only blends existing concepts. Imagination can be a preview of new things. The mental image appears first, and needs only to be mobilized by desire for something new to manifest in your world.

It is not possible to achieve psychic autonomy and self-determination without self-discipline. Our resolve sometimes falls short. It is difficult to do things that are not rewarded by immediate pleasure. This is where the imagination must lend a hand to the will. It permits us to anticipate and believe that we will be recompensed for our efforts, sooner or later. We learned aspects of this during childhood and adolescence, and it was not always easy.

It is possible to strengthen willpower by practicing things that have clear benefit. For example:

- wake up fifteen minutes earlier in the morning to practice some of the book's exercises that are valuable to your inner balance and existence;

- choose fruit in place of commercial desserts, which bring no vital element to your organism;
- read a book or journal that enriches you mentally or spiritually; it is better than sitting on the couch in front of a television; and
- take up some form of regular physical exercise or stretching routine to keep your body in a dynamic condition.

We often maintain the belief that we lack the time to give over to such activities. With an honest assessment, we realize that it is not difficult to find a few minutes during the day, if we take some time away from nonessential pursuits, those whose effects and satisfaction are more ephemeral.

A proposed sequence is set out in the calendar on the next page. Little by little you will become habituated to paying attention to your inner world, on different levels, and at different moments in your day. In a fairly short time, you may find yourself, quite out of the blue, discovering fresh perceptions, new points of view, and catching glimpses of a more positive life.

Feel free to adapt this program to methods that are already familiar to you, to your own possibilities, and to life circumstances. As with so many endeavors, regularity is the key to success. It is better to practice five minutes every day than an hour once in a while. Excessive enthusiasm at the start risks a rapid decline.

Depending on your temperament and the time you truly wish to devote to your physical and spiritual health, commit yourself to practice only the exercises you like best. You can certainly extend the time suggested for each step. The important thing is that you do something for yourself towards gaining freedom and vitality.

Any difficulties at the beginning are sure to fade. The initial push to get started will disappear, replaced by a new enthusiasm.

The practices laid out are founded on proven and solid methods. I have invented nothing. Whether it be the techniques or notions about our emotional or mental makeup, I have simply collected various findings and experiences, drawn from ancient and modern sources. My main contribution is to have gathered the information into a coherent whole to benefit those who have found this approach helpful in overcoming current difficulties, in order that they may participate in a fuller and more serene life.

This book is dedicated to all those who have been wronged in some way, suffer daily, and are imprisoned by stress and anxiety. Stress is a prison whose doors are open—cross the threshold!

Training calendar

Week 1

Evening of day one
Exercise 1: Observation (page 59)

Each evening after day one
Exercise 2: Coherent breathing (page 61)

Week 2

Every morning
Exercise 3: Physiological cohesion (page 62)

Use this exercise whenever you feel the inclination. (See indications given in the exercise.)

Each evening
Exercise 2: Coherent breathing (page 61)

Week 3

Every morning
Exercise 4: Cardiac coherence (page 62)

Each evening
Exercise 4: Cardiac coherence (page 62)
Exercise 9: Visualization (page 71)

Week 4

Every morning
Exercise 4: Cardiac coherence (page 62)

Each evening
Exercise 4: Cardiac coherence (page 62)
Exercise 10: The safe place (page 74)

Week 5

Every morning
Exercise 4: Cardiac coherence (page 62)

First two evenings
Exercise 5: Observation (repeat version) (page 66)
Exercise 11: Emotional control (page 76)

This exercise can then be used whenever necessary.

Following evenings
Exercise 4: Cardiac coherence (page 62)
Exercise 12: The Buddha smile (page 78)

This exercise can be used whenever necessary.

Week 6

Every morning
Exercise 4: Cardiac coherence (page 62)

Each evening
Exercise 6: Interlude and sound (page 66)
Exercise 15: Developing attention (page 96)

Week 7

Every morning
Exercise 4: Cardiac coherence (page 62)

Each evening
Exercise 7: Pause on inhalation (page 67)
Exercise 14: Relaxation (page 89)

Week 8

Every morning
Exercise 4: Cardiac coherence (page 62)

Each evening
Exercise 7: Pause on inhalation (page 67)

Each evening, but alternate between Exercise 13 and 14
Exercise 13: Unfolding desires (page 81), the first phase only.
Exercise 14: Relaxation (page 89)

Practice this exercise whenever, and for as long as you wish (three times a week, for example).

Week 9

Every morning
Exercise 3: Physiological coherence (page 62)

Each evening
Exercise 8: Pause on exhalation (page 67)
Exercise 13: Unfolding desire (page 81), second phase

Week 10

Daily, ideally morning and evening, for an indefinite period
Practice coherent breathing for several minutes at a time, finding your personal rhythm that has been established over weeks of practice. This breathing rhythm will become more and more natural and instinctive, whenever you find yourself feeling calm.

Several evenings during the week
Alternate the following practices:
Exercise 9: Visualization (page 71), assessment
Exercise 10: The safe place (page 74)
Exercise 15: Developing attention (page 96)

Week 11

Every morning
Exercise 16: Complexes: activation and de-activation (page 99)

Each evening
Exercise 17: Positive attitude (page 101)

Week 12

Every morning
Exercise 16: Complexes: activation and de-activation (page 99)

Each evening
Exercise 17: Positive attitude (page 101)

One evening during the week
Exercise 11: Emotional control (page 76)

Week 13

Every morning
Exercise 16: Complexes: activation and de-activation (page 99)

Each evening
Exercise 17: Positive attitude (page 101)

One or two evenings during the week
Review Exercise 13: Unfolding desire (page 81)

Week 14

Every other morning
Exercise 16: Complexes: activation and de-activation (page 99)

Each evening
Exercise 18: Concentration (page 103)

One or two evenings during the week
Review Exercise 10: The safe place (page 74)

Week 15

Every other morning
Exercise 16: Complex de-activation and activation (page 99)

Every other evening, alternating with every other morning
Exercise 18: Concentration (page 103)

One or two evenings during the week
Review of Exercise 12: The Buddha smile (page 78)

Week 16

Every other morning
Exercise 16: Complex de-activation and activation (page 99)

Every other morning, alternating with mornings
Exercise 18: Concentration (page 103)

One or two evenings during the week
Review of Exercise 13: Unfolding desire (page 81)

And afterwards?

Your life is your own. Take stock of what you have gained from these exercises.

Some readers have adapted the suggested program to suit their capacities better. The calendar represents an idealized version of practice, after all. Relative to the time and effort you have put in, do you feel that changes in the quality of your life, including the benefits to physiological, emotional, and mental equilibrium, are the best for which you can hope?

Depending on your answer, it is up to you to find your own rhythm, and design a more perfect program made up of the exercises you particularly enjoy. This process may awaken an interest in similar practices, or lead you to pursue additional sources of inner fulfillment and development.

This is my wish for you.

Observations and Progress

Below are a series of questions that you can complete when you first start using these exercises. Note the day and date when you first answer the questions. Then after one month, three months, and six months, answer these questions again. See how you are progressing.

Do you breathe in and out with equal ease?

1. Starting Date _____

2. After one month _____

3. After three months _____

4. After six months _____

Which parts of the breathing cycle seem more mobile?

1. Starting Date _____

2. After one month _____

3. After three months _____

4. After six months _____

Does your belly inflate as your chest expands?

    1. Starting Date _____

    2. After one month _____

    3. After three months _____

    4. After six months _____

Do you breathe through your nose, mouth, or both at once?

    1. Starting Date _____

    2. After one month _____

    3. After three months _____

    4. After six months _____

Is your respiration deep or shallow?

   1. Starting Date _____

   2. After one month _____

   3. After three months _____

   4. After six months _____

In daily life, at what point do you feel unbalanced by your emotions?

   1. Starting Date _____

   2. After one month _____

   3. After three months _____

   4. After six months _____

Did you succeed in remaining focused on your breath, or did your thoughts have a tendency to disperse, follow their own path or wander towards some current preoccupation?

1. Starting Date _____

2. After one month _____

3. After three months _____

4. After six months _____

Relative to the time and effort you have put in, do you feel that changes in the quality of your life, including the benefits to physiological, emotional, and mental equilibrium, are the best that can be hoped for?

1. Starting Date _____

2. After one month _____

3. After three months _____

4. After six months _____

Now that you have some experience with breath, through practicing the cardiac coherence exercises, return to passively observing your breath, as first instructed. What differences do you notice, if any, from the initial experience? If you have jotted down your first impressions, it will be easy to see your headway.

1. Starting Date _____

2. After one month _____

3. After three months _____

4. After six months _____

What are your preferred sensory systems for visualization?

1. Date _____

    Visual _____

    Kinesthetic _____

    Auditory _____

    Smell and Taste _____

How can we manage our emotions and gradually elevate the nature of emotions that inhabit us? Ideally, we would never find ourselves having to deal with being emotionally overwhelmed. Does this seem impossible?

    1. Starting Date _____

    2. After one month _____

    3. After three months _____

    4. After six months _____

How do you come back into balance and reconnect with yourself, after an emotion has thrown you askew?

    1. Starting Date _____

    2. After one month _____

    3. After three months _____

    4. After six months _____

What negative autosuggestions can you switch to positive autosuggestions that enhance your well-being, liberty, and creativity of purpose?

    1. Starting Date _____

    2. After one month _____

    3. After three months _____

    4. After six months _____

Bibliography

Alexander Franz, *La médecine psychosomatique,* Petite Bibliothèque Payot, 1962.

Assagioli Roberto, *Psychosynthèse,* Épi, 1983.

Bailey Alice, *Lettres sur la méditation occulte,* Lucis Trust, 1922.

Bercot Michel, Cœur et Énergétique. Les structures énergétiques du vivant, Opéra éditions, 1999.

Besant Annie, (1901), *Le pouvoir de la pensée,* Adyar, 2000.

Besant Annie, (1902), *Les lois de la vie supérieure,* Adyar, 1994.

Blofeld John, Le bouddhisme tantrique du Tibet, Seuil, 1976.

Bossy Jean, Anatomie Clinique, 4 – *Neuro-anatomie,* Springer-Verlag, 1990.

Bourret Paul et Louis René, *Anatomie du système nerveux central,* L'expansion scientifique française, troisième édition, 1986.

Calais-Germain Blandine, *Respiration anatomie – geste respiratoire,* DésIris, 2005.

Cancelliere Vito Mariano, de Riba Francis, *La réponse apaisante au stress,* Jouvence, 2003.

Caporossi Roger, Le système neuro-végétatif et ses troubles fonctionnels, Éditions de Verlaque, 1994.

Changeux Jean-Pierre, *L'homme neuronal,* Fayard, «Pluriel», 1983.

Damasio Antonio, *L'erreur de Descartes,* Odile Jacob, 1995.

Damasio Antonio, *Le sentiment même de soi,* Odile Jacob, 1999.

Dantzer Robert, *L'illusion psychosomatique,* Odile Jacob, 1989.

Danner DD1, Snowdon DA, Friesen WV., Positive emotions in early life and longevity: findings from the nun study, J Pers Soc Psychol. 2001 May;80(5):804-13.

Erickson Milton, *L'hypnose thérapeutique,* ESF, 1986.

F. Gregory Ashby, Alice M. Isen, A Neuropsychological Theory of

Positive Affect and Its Influence on Cognition, Psychological Review 1999, Vol. 106, No. 3. 529-550.

Freud Sigmund, (1915), *Métapsychologie*, Gallimard, 1968.

Freud Sigmund, *La technique psychanalytique*, P.U.F., 1953.

Freud Sigmund, *Le moi et les mécanismes de défense*, P.U.F., 1949.

Gazzaniga Michael, Ivry Richard, Mangun George, *Neurosciences cognitives*. La biologie de l'esprit, De Boeck Université, «Neurosciences et Cognition», 2001, traduction de la première édition américaine.

Haley Jay, *Un thérapeute hors du commun: Milton H. Erickson*, Desclée de Brouwer, 1984.

Heart rate variability – Standards of measurement, physiological interpretation, and clinical use – Task Force of The European Society of Cardiology and The North American Society of Pacing and Electrophysiology, European Heart Journal (1996) 17, 354–381

Houdé Olivier, Mazoyer Bernard, Tzourio-Mazoyer Nathalie, *Cerveau et psychologie*, P.U.F., «Premier cycle», 2002.

Israël Lucien, *Cerveau droit*, cerveau gauche, Plon, 1995.

Jung Carl Gustav, *Dialectique du Moi et de l'inconscient*, Gallimard, 1964 (1ère éd. 1933).

Jung Carl Gustav, *Psychologie de l'inconscient*, Georg éditeur, 1993 (1ère éd. 1952).

Jung Carl Gustav, *Types psychologiques*, Georg éditeur, 1991 (1ère éd. 1950).

Jung Carl Gustav, *La guérison psychologique*, Georg éditeur, 1993 (1ère éd. 1953).

Jung Carl Gustav, *L'énergétique psychique*, Georg éditeur, 1993 (1ère éd. 1956).

Kamieniecki Hanna, *Histoire de la psychosomatique*, P.U.F., 1994.

Lama Anagarika Govinda, *Les fondements de la mystique tibétaine*, Albin Michel, 1960.

Lao-Tseu, *Tao Te King*, Albin Michel, 1984.

Laurency Henry, *La Pierre des Sages*, Opéra éditions, 2005.

Lavorel Pierre, *Psychologie et cerveau*, Presses Universitaires de Lyon, 1991.

Lôo Pierre, Lôo Henri et Galinowski André, Le stress permanent, Masson, 1999.

Louise H. Phillips, Rebecca Bull, Ewan Adams, and Lisa Fraser, Positive Mood and Executive Function: Evidence From Stroop and Fluency Tasks, Emotion 2002, Vol. 2, No. 1, 12–22.

Marty Pierre, Les mouvements individuels de vie et de mort, Payot, 1976.

Marty Pierre, L'ordre psychosomatique, Payot, 1980.

Mc Craty R., Barrios-ChopplinB., Rozman D., AtkinsonM., Watkins A.D., The impact of a new emotional self-management program on stress, emotions, Heart rate variability, DHEA and Cortisol, Integrative Physiological and Behavioral Science, Vol. 33, N°2. April - June 1998.

Millenson J.R., Le corps et l'esprit, DésIris, 1998.

Muller Martin, Introduction à l'ontologie – Vers l'actualisation de l'homme total, © Martin Muller, 1974.

Oschman James L., "Energy medicine, the scientific basis." Churchill Livingston, 2000.

Porges S.W., International Journal of Psychophysiology 42 (2001) 123-146

Porges S.W., The polyvagal perspective, Biol Psychol. 2007 Feb; 74(2): 116–143.

Rossi Ernest, Psychobiologie de la guérison, Le Souffle d'Or, 2002.

Roustang François, La fin de la plainte, Odile Jacob, 2000.

Servan-Schreiber David, Guérir le stress, l'anxiété et la dépression sans médicaments ni psychanalyse, Robert Laffont, 2003.

Tortora Gerard, Grabowski Bogdan, Principes d'anatomie et de physiologie, De Boeck université, 3e édition, 2005.

Villemain Françoise, Stress et Immunologie, P.U.F., «Nodules», 1989.

Vincent Jean-Didier, Biologie des passions, Odile Jacob, nouvelle édition, 1994.

Vincent Jean-Didier, La chair et le diable, Odile Jacob, 1996.

Watts Alan, L'esprit du Zen, Dangles, 1976.

Watzlawick Paul, Wiener-Renucci Jeanne, Bansard Denis, Le langage du changement, Seuil, «Points», 1980.

Watzlawick Paul, L'invention de la réalité, Seuil, «Points essais», 1988.

‖BARRAL
‖PRODUCTIONS

Your source for quality educational materials.

Titles also available:

For General Public:

Understanding Messages of Your Joints

Understanding the Messages of Your Body

An Answer to Your Pain

Your Inner Physician and You

For Healthcare Professionals:

Manual Therapy for the Peripheral Nerves

Manual Therapy for the Cranial Nerves

Manual Therapy for the Prostate

Visceral Vascular Manipulation

New Manual Articular Approach; Upper Extremity

New Manual Articular Approach; Lower Extremity

www.Barralinstitute.com